DATE DUE

DEMCO 38-296

INJURY PREVENTION
FOR THE ELDERLY

Recent Titles in
Bibliographies and Indexes in Gerontology

INJURY PREVENTION FOR THE ELDERLY

A Research Guide

Compiled by
Bonnie L. Walker

Bibliographies and Indexes in Gerontology, Number 30
Erdman B. Palmore, Series Adviser

GREENWOOD PRESS
Westport, Connecticut • London

Library of Congress Cataloging-in-Publication Data

Walker, Bonnie L.
    Injury prevention for the elderly : a research guide / compiled by
Bonnie L. Walker.
        p. cm.—(Bibliographies and indexes in gerontology, ISSN
0743–7560 ; no. 30)
    Includes bibliographical references and index.
    ISBN 0–313–29670–7 (alk. paper)
    1. Aged—Accidents—Prevention—Bibliography. 2. Accidents—
Prevention—Bibliography. 3. Aged—Wounds and injuries—
Bibliography. 4. Abused aged—Bibliography. 5. Falls (Accidents)
in old age—Bibliography. I. Title. II. Series.
Z7164.04W28   1995
[HV675.7]
016.3631'00846—dc20   95–32989

British Library Cataloguing in Publication Data is available.

Library of Congress Catalog Card Number: 95–32989
ISSN: 0–313–29670–7
ISSN: 0743–7560

First published in 1995

Greenwood Press, 88 Post Road West, Westport, CT 06881
An imprint of Greenwood Publishing Group, Inc.

Printed in the United States of America

∞™

The paper used in this book complies with the
Permanent Paper Standard issued by the National
Information Standards Organization (Z39.48–1984).

10 9 8 7 6 5 4 3 2

Portions of this book were prepared pursuant to the Centers for Disease Control Grant Number 1R43CE00051-01. Some of the references related to problem use of alcohol were obtained
pursuant to the National Institute on Alcoholism and Alcohol Abuse Project Number
N43AA4212. The statements and conclusions herein are those of Bonnie Walker & Associates, Inc., and do not necessarily reflect the views or policies of the sponsoring agencies.

To my parents, Ray and Alice Theuret

Contents

Series Foreword

The annotated bibliographies in this series provide answers to the fundamental question, "What is known?" Their purpose is simple, yet profound: to provide comprehensive reviews and references for the work done in various fields of gerontology. They are based on the fact that it is no longer possible for anyone to comprehend the vast body of research and writing in even one sub-specialty without years of work.

This fact has become true only in recent years. When I was an undergraduate (Class of '52) I think no one at Duke had even heard of gerontology. Almost no one in the world was identified as a gerontologist. Now there are over 6,000 professional members of the Gerontological Society of America. When I was an undergraduate, there were no courses in gerontology. Now there are thousands of courses offered by most major (and many minor) colleges and universities. When I was an undergraduate, there was only one gerontological journal (the *Journal of Gerontology*, begun in 1945). Now there are over forty professional journals and several dozen books in gerontology published each year.

The reasons for this dramatic growth are well known: the dramatic increase in numbers of aged, the shift from family to public responsibility for the security and care of the elderly. The recognition of aging as a "social problem," and the growth of science in general. It is less well known that this explosive growth in knowledge has developed the need for new solutions to the old problem of comprehending and "keeping up" with a field of knowledge. The old indexes and library card catalogues have become increasingly inadequate for the job. On-line computer indexes and abstracts are one solution but make no evaluative selections nor organize sources logically as is done here. The annotated bibliographies in our series are also more widely available than on-line computer indexes.

This bibliography is designed to maximize ease of access. One can use it in four different ways: begin with the chapter dealing with the injury of interest, begin with the index of topics, or begin with the index of authors.

In the past, the "review of literature" has often been haphazard and was rarely comprehensive, because of the large investment of time (and money) that would be required by a truly comprehensive review. Now, using these bibliographies, researchers, teachers, students, and others concerned with a topic can be more confident that they are not missing important previous literature and reports; they can be more confident that they are not duplicating past efforts and "reinventing the wheel." It may well become standard and expected practice for researchers to consult such bibliographies, even before they start their research.

In recent decades there has been a growing interest in injury prevention for the elderly. This is attested to by the 621 references in this bibliography. It has become more and more evident that elders are at increased risk of suffering injuries and that many of these injuries could be prevented.

The main purpose of this bibliography is to provide information that could be used in an injury prevention training program for people who care for elders in long-term care facilities and in the community. However, it should also be useful to anyone concerned with injury prevention among elders, whether they are elders themselves, relatives or friends of elders, health care professionals, gerontologists, administrators, public policy professionals, or researchers.

The author has done an outstanding job of covering the literature and organizing it into easily accessible form. This bibliography is unusual in the large number of references it contains and the extensive information that is contained in each reference.

So it is with great pleasure that we add this bibliography to our series. We believe you will find this volume to be the most useful, comprehensive, and easily accessible reference work in its field. I will appreciate any comments you care to send me.

Erdman B. Palmore

Preface

The purpose of this literature review was to provide information that could be used to develop an injury prevention training program curriculum for people who care for the elderly in long-term care facilities as well as in the community.

Unintentional injury is one of the leading causes of death to elderly people. The most common types of fatal injuries to people ages 60 and over are motor vehicle crashes, falls, fires and burns, surgical and medical complications, poisoning, suffocation by ingestion (choking), and drowning. Other types of accidental death that disproportionately affect elderly people are adverse effects of heat and cold (hyperthermia and hypothermia), pedestrian accidents, malnutrition, and food poisoning. Older people also suffer both injury and death from physical, emotional, and financial abuse and neglect. Suicide also disproportionately affects the elderly. Problem use of alcohol is interrelated to several types of injuries, especially falls, medication problems, motor vehicle crashes, suicide, and drowning, but it is also a problem with its own characteristics, causes, and potential for intervention. Understanding each of these problems, their causes, and model prevention techniques can lead health care providers and policymakers to adopt practices that will reduce these needless deaths and injuries.

The injury areas that are included in this book were identified as a result of a literature search and through discussions with experts in gerontology, injury prevention, in specialized fields such as alcohol research and pharmacology, and people who provide care to older people. The process of locating the most important and most current research was circular and involved literature searches, discussions of findings, more literature searches, and more discussions.

Many references were located from searches of the Expanded Academic Index, ERIC, Medline, and Articles1st. The AAA Foundation for Traffic Safety provided its research literature related to motor vehicle crashes and the elderly. *Alcoholism and Aging: An Annotated Bibliography and Review* by Nancy J. Osgood, Helen E. Wood, and Iris A. Parham published by Greenwood Press was an important source of research related to problem use of alcohol. Dr. Osgood also provided assistance in locating many of the resources related to elderly suicide. Dr. Jean Wyman guided us to many of the articles related to falls; Dr. Ilene Zuckerman provided copies of several important studies related to medications. Dr. Frederic Blow provided information about most current research in developing alcohol screening instruments for the elderly. The National Clearinghouse on Alcohol and Drug Information (NCADI) provided a literature search on problem use of alcohol among the elderly and substance abuse assessment instruments. Bonnie Walker & Associates, Inc., used its own extensive reference library to locate information about burns and scalds. The National Fire Protection Association provided many items related to that topic from its research collection.

References selected for each section were those which provided information about prevalence, risk factors, specific causes, and prevention techniques related to that injury area. The articles included provided information that is useful to people who care for the elderly, who conduct research to better understand aging and elderly people, or who supervise or train people who care for the elderly.

The first chapter of this book includes references which address injury prevention in general or more than one injury class. The remaining chapters are arranged alphabetically by injury class. A summary of the findings related to each injury prevention topic is presented at the beginning of each chapter. Resource materials, such as videos or curriculum guides related to specific topics, are included in the related chapters.

Acknowledgments

The following individuals assisted the author at various stages of this project in locating and selecting materials that are included in this book: Edward F. Ansello, Ph.D., Virginia Center on Aging, Medical College of Virginia; Kenneth H. Beck, Ph.D., Department of Health Education, University of Maryland; Frederic Blow, Ph.D., University of Michigan; Peter Lamy, Ph.D., School of Pharmacy, University of Maryland at Baltimore; Nancy J. Osgood, Ph.D., Department of Gerontology and Sociology, Medical College of Virginia; Jean F. Wyman, RN, Ph.D., School of Nursing, Medical College of Virginia; Ilene H. Zuckerman, Pharm.D., School of Pharmacy, University of Maryland at Baltimore.

The following individuals assisted the author in conducting the research and in editing the text: Cheryl L. Fischer, Janice Torry, and April L. Walker. The author is especially appreciative of Lise M. Holliker's help in editing many of the entries, locating articles in libraries, and preparing the final manuscript.

1

General Injury Prevention

Unintentional injuries account for a large number of fatalities to people ages 65 and over. Injury prevention for the elderly has been the focus of only a few studies. In most cases researchers focus on specific injury classes. Falls, medications, motor vehicle crashes, and problem use of alcohol have stimulated the greatest number of articles. Elder abuse, a problem area which includes many other types of injury, has also engendered a great deal of interest by researchers. While choking is a leading cause of death among the very old (ages 90 and over), few studies have been conducted on that topic. Other injury areas that affect a significant number of elderly people are related to exposure to heat or cold, drowning, pedestrian accidents, food poisoning, and suicide. Finally, there is malnutrition, a problem often suffered by older people which causes preventable bodily harm. Chapter 1 lists books and articles about the prevalence of major kinds of injuries including incidence among the elderly, risk factors, prevention research, and the cost of injuries. These publications address injuries across types rather than a single class of injuries.

001 Abdellah, Faye G., & Moore, Steven R. (Eds.). (March 20-23, 1988). *Surgeon General's Workshop: Health promotion and aging.* Washington, DC: U. S. Department of Health and Human Services Public Health Service.

This book is a report of the proceedings of the 1988 Surgeon General's Workshop. The sessions focused on health promotion activities and agendas for older Americans. The workshop also included working groups of experts in the areas of alcohol, dental (oral) health, physical fitness and exercise, injury prevention, medications, mental health, nutrition, preventive health services, and smoking cessation. The working groups made several recommendations for action and further research in each area.

002   *Accident prevention.* (1991). Gaithersburg, MD: National Institute on Aging.

This pamphlet gives accident prevention suggestions for the elderly. Because the elderly are at higher risk for injury and death from accidents, taking steps to prevent those accidents is important. The accidents described include falls, burns, and motor vehicle and pedestrian accidents. The pamphlet also provides resources for further information on accident prevention.

003   **American Red Cross, & Handal, Kathleen A. (1992).** *The American Red Cross first aid and safety handbook.* **Boston, MA: Little, Brown and Company.**

This book discusses basic emergency procedures, first aid, and injury prevention techniques. Emergency situations are described with detailed instructions for giving emergency care and contacting appropriate medical help. The first aid section describes 30 types of injuries, giving the most common signs and symptoms as well as first aid techniques to help stabilize the condition until medical help is provided. The last section discusses personal and family safety, giving lists of ways that the reader can eliminate home, fire, disaster, outdoor, sports, water, and motor vehicle safety hazards. The book also includes a list of resource organizations and available American Red Cross first aid courses.

004   **Baker, Susan P. (1975). Determinants of injury and opportunities for intervention.** *American Journal of Epidemiology, 101*(2), 98-102.

This article explores the reasons why some groups of people experience more injuries than others. For example, elderly people have a high rate of pedestrian fatalities. This is not necessarily a direct result of age, but may result from age-associated decreases in an elderly person's ability to perceive moving cars or respond quickly and appropriately in an emergency. Interventions should be directed at the risk factors of the group of people, rather than at the people themselves. The article discusses four categories of countermeasures: modification of the environment; perceptual aids, training and education; strengthening the individual who would otherwise be injured; and emergency response systems and medical treatment. Modification of the environment has the greatest potential as an effective intervention because it does not rely on human cooperation or behavior to prevent injuries.

005   Baker, Susan P., O'Neill, Brian, Ginsburg, Marvin J., & Li, Guohua. (1992). *The injury fact book*. New York: Oxford University Press.

    This book gives an overview of injury and injury mortality in the United States and discusses the intentional or unintentional nature of these injuries. Categories of injuries include suicide, homicide, sports and recreation injuries, vehicle-related injuries, occupational injuries, falls, firearm-related injuries, fires and burns, drowning, asphyxiation by choking and suffocation, and poisoning. Each category is discussed according to the place of injury, the victims of the injury by age, gender, race, and per capita income, geographic differences, historical trends, and preventive measures.

006   Bever, David L. (1992). *Safety: A personal focus*. St. Louis, MO: Mosby-Year Book, Inc.

    This book, which was designed for use as a introductory safety course textbook, discusses how people can protect themselves from injuries and injury hazards. The author defines safety and describes safety measures for many specific areas and types of hazards: homes, fires, personal protection and firearms, motor vehicles and pedestrian safety, the workplace, natural and man-made disasters, recreational activities, and schools. The book also discusses age-specific safety topics, including hypothermia, pedestrian accidents, and falls among the elderly.

007   Christoffel, Tom. (1989). The role of law in reducing injury. *Law, Medicine & Health Care, 17*(1), 7-16.

    This article discusses the recommendations of injury prevention experts from a legal point of view. The three most often recommended strategies to prevent injuries are to persuade persons at risk to alter their behavior for increased self protection, to adopt laws or administrative rules requiring individual behavior change, and to provide automatic protection through improved product design. Opponents of the second strategy (injury prevention laws) propose that the laws don't work to prevent injuries, that such laws pose too much of a restriction on individual liberty, and that the cost of enforcing the laws is too high. These objections should be either validated or refuted by future research. The author suggests that laws can only be an effective means of injury prevention if the general public understands and supports the need for them.

008   **Committee on Trauma Research. (1986).** *Injury in America: A Continuing Public Health Problem.* **Washington, DC: National Academy Press.**
       This book reviews the subject of injury epidemiology, prevention, treatment, and research. The authors illustrate the current magnitude of the injury problem in the United States with results of existing studies, and give specific recommendations for further research. General methods of injury prevention are described, with their specific applications to different types of injuries. The authors also review current funding for injury research and give recommendations for improved administration and funding.

009   *Cost of injury in the United States: A report to Congress 1989.* **(1989). Atlanta, GA: Centers for Disease Control.**
       This report discusses the incidence and cost of injury in the United States. It includes 1985 data on the number and rate of persons injured by gender, age, and class of injury, by cause and class of injury, and by intent and class of injury. It also includes information on injury morbidity losses by age and gender, by gender and cause, and mortality losses by age and gender, and by gender and cause.

010   **Department of Health and Human Services. (1992).** *Position Papers from The Third National Injury Control Conference.* **Washington, DC: U. S. Government Printing Office.**
       This book discusses the prevalence and prevention of major injuries in the United States. The topics include motor vehicle injury prevention, prevention of violence and injuries due to violence, home and leisure injury prevention, occupational injury prevention, trauma care systems, acute care treatment, and rehabilitation of people with injuries. Each topic is discussed according to present statistics, future goals, and plans to implement those goals.

011   **Dijkhuis, Hannah, Zwerling, Craig, Parrish, Gib, Bennett, Thomas, & Kemper, Han C. G. (March 15, 1994). Medical**

Examiner data in injury surveillance: A comparison with death certificates. *American Journal of Epidemiology, 139*(6), 637-643.

This study compared medical examiner databases from a two-year period to actual death certificates to determine whether injury epidemiology studies based on these databases can be accurate. Medical examiners reported 68.7% of fatal injuries, which included 36.9% of fall fatalities, 79.2% of transportation fatalities, 82.6% of intentional fatalities, and 57.3% of other external causes of death. Women's injury-related deaths, as well as elderly injury deaths, were less likely to be reported by medical examiners. Among the elderly, falls and transportation fatalities were investigated less often, and intentional injuries were investigated most often. The authors conclude that medical examiner data, although detailed, contain an underreported number of injury deaths, and suggest that these data (especially among certain groups) should be compared with death certificates when researching injury epidemiology.

012   Duffy, Mary E., & MacDonald, Ellen. (August, 1990). Determinants of functional health of older persons. *The Gerontologist, 30*(4), 503-509.

This study used several markers of functional health to determine which health promotion activities were associated with better functioning in the elderly (ages 65 and over). Subjects were 179 elderly men and women from southeast Texas. Tests of health locus of control, self-esteem, health-promoting lifestyle, and health perceptions were compared to the results of a functional health assessment. The findings indicate significant relationships between certain demographic variables, control of health, self-esteem, health promotion activities, and health status. The authors suggest that exercise and nutrition as health promotion activities may be critical to functional health in this population.

013   Eggert, Russell W., & Parkinson, Michael D. (September 7, 1994). Preventive medicine and health reform: Improving physician education, training, and practice. *Journal of the American Medical Association, 272*(9), 688-693.

This article discusses the issues related to the current need for and shortage of preventive medicine physicians. The leading causes of death in the United States—tobacco, diet and activity patterns, alcohol, diseases, firearms, sexual behavior, motor vehicles, and illicit drugs—can be attacked through preventive medicine and interventions. Current funding, however, tends to focus on high-tech interventions that have less clinical benefit than other interventions that have already been proven effective. The authors recommend that better training of preventive medicine physicians will provide more effective research and intervention in the causes of preventable deaths.

014   Heckler, Margaret M. (March-April, 1985). Health promotion for older Americans. *Public Health Reports, 100*(2), 225-230.

This article describes a Department of Health and Human Services initiative to promote health and fitness among older Americans. Studies have shown that the elderly are extremely health-conscious and are willing to adopt habits that will maintain good health. The initiative is focused on six areas: fitness-exercise, nutrition, safe and proper use of drugs and alcohol, accident prevention, other preventive services, and smoking cessation. The initiative includes distributing printed information, providing nutritious meals for the elderly, initiating a Food and Drug Administration consumer education program, continuing Centers for Disease Control programs on accident prevention, creating an Alzheimer's disease task force, and a media campaign of health promotion for the elderly. At least three national health and senior citizens organizations are working closely with HHS agencies on the initiative. The author also describes efforts to encourage growing health maintenance organizations that promote health and prevention for their Medicare members, and suggest that continuing government and private sector research into health promotion will improve health and life satisfaction for elderly people.

015   Jenkins, Antoinette, Corby, Nancy H., Moore, Julie, & Small, Arnold M. (Eds.). (1975). *Safety for the elderly: A selected bibliography.* Los Angeles, CA: University of Southern California Press.

This bibliography lists approximately 300 titles representing a search of the literature from 1955 to 1975 with brief annotations divided into the following topics: community safety, general safety, home safety, institutional safety, physiological research, statistics, and vehicle accidents.

016   King, Amy Suzanne. (1989). Accidents claim 96,000 lives, but rate declining for some types. *Journal of the American Medical Association, 262*(16), 2195.

The author uses accident statistics from 1988 to describe accident and injury trends in the United States. Nearly half of all accidental deaths during this year occurred during traffic accidents. Home accidents were the second most common, for which the elderly and young children were at highest risk. Nearly 40% of falls resulting in death occurred at home, and more than 50% of these fall deaths involved the elderly (ages 75 and over). Residential fires were responsible for 75% of all burn fatalities. Other common accidental deaths resulted from poisoning, workplace hazards, and drownings.

017   Levy, David B., Hanlon, Dennis P., & Townsend, Ricard N. (August, 1993). Geriatric trauma. *Clinics in Geriatric Medicine, 9*(3), 601-620.

This article is a review of the epidemiology, evaluation, and management of elderly trauma victims. The epidemiology of injuries suffered by the elderly is different than for younger groups, and elderly people are more likely to die from less serious injuries than younger people. Because the causes and physiological effects of injuries are different for the elderly, the management and prevention of these injuries should be different than measures used for younger people.

018   Mahoney, Cheryl. (March, 1991). Return to independence: Lessons from a hospital long-term care unit. *American Journal of Nursing, 91*(3), 44-48.

The author describes a program used to determine whether hospitalized elderly could, through an interim long-term care program, return home rather than enter a nursing home. The program, used at a New York hospital, targeted the chronic illnesses and general health problems of those elderly deemed unable to maintain independence as a result of hospitalization. During the five years of this program, 183 of 267 patients demonstrated enough improvement to return home, 75 entered nursing homes needing a lower level of supervision, and only nine needed extended nursing home care. The authors estimate that all 267 patients would all otherwise have been placed in nursing homes. The long-term care unit was closed in 1989 due to insufficient funds.

019   Mayer, Jeffrey P., Taylor, Jeffrey R., & Thrush, John C. (December, 1990). Exploratory cluster analysis of behavioral risks for chronic disease and injury: Implications for tailoring

health promotion services. *Journal of Community Health, 15*(6), 377-389.

The authors used telephone surveys to identify groups of people with similar behavioral risks for different types of injuries. Four groups were identified: middle age hypertensives, young achievers, risk takers, and poverty multiple risk. The middle age hypertensives were generally older in age, overweight, and showing some form of hypertension, but were generally cautious in other areas such as low levels of smoking, high frequency of exercise, use of seatbelts, and low levels of drinking. The young achievers showed high frequency of exercise, thinness, below average age and level of hypertension, and above average education and income. Despite the low risks for this group, the young achievers had a high prevalence of alcohol consumption and drinking and driving. More than 75% of this group were classified as acute drinkers. The risk takers were characterized by high levels of smoking and low frequency of exercise, as well as below average education and income. Almost 50% of this group were smokers, and over 85% said they did not exercise regularly. The poverty multiple risk group was characterized by hypertension, low use of seatbelts, above average age, and greatly below average education and income. This group had the highest percentage of elderly people, women, and minorities. These cluster groups may be used to target health promotion programs at the specific risks for each group.

020   McCaig, Linda F. (March 2, 1994). National Hospital Ambulatory Medical Care Survey: 1992 emergency department summary. *Advance Data, 245,* 1-12.

This report lists the most common cause of injuries treated in emergency rooms in 1992. These causes included accidental falls (26.6%), motor vehicle accidents (14.3%), homicide and assault (5.4%), accidents due to natural and environmental factors (4.8%), accidents caused by submersion, suffocation, and foreign bodies (3.6%), other road vehicle accidents (2.2%), surgical and medical procedures (1.4%), adverse effects of drugs (1.3%), accidental poisoning by drugs (1.2%), poisoning by other solid and liquid substances, gases, and vapors (0.7%), suicide (0.6%), and fire and flames (0.4%), and other accidents (35.8%). People ages 65 and over accounted for 2.7% of all injury-related emergency visits. The most common reasons for visiting an emergency room were stomach and abdominal pain (5.5%), chest pain (5.2%), fever (4.1%), headache (2.8%), cuts on the upper body (2.6%), shortness of breath (2.3%), cough (2.2%), back symptoms (2.2%), throat problems (2.2%), vomiting (2.1%), or other pain (2.0%). Other symptoms accounted for less than 2% each.

021   **Mercer, Susan O. (1983). Consequences of institutionalization of the aged. In Jordan I. Kosberg, Ed.** *Abuse and maltreatment of the elderly: Causes and interventions* **(pp. 84-103). Boston: John Wright • PSG Inc.**

This essay reviews the impact of institutionalization on an elderly person, particularly the loss of control and choice as well as the concomitant effects of learned helplessness with relocation to a long-term care facility. The author describes the characteristics of nursing home residents primarily from data gathered in the 1970s. Approximately 5% to 15% are disabled by deafness, blindness, or serious illnesses, and about 50% require help with activities of daily living. About one-fourth to one-third are confused most of the time. The average time of residence is two years. Most of these residents, 56%, come from their own homes, 31% come from hospitals, and 13% come from other nursing homes. Within this population, 88% are ages 65 and over, with a median age of 82. Women outnumber men three to one. Men are younger and more likely to be divorced or never married. Blacks comprise only 4% of the nursing home population, despite making up 11% of the elderly population. As a result of living in an environment which is essentially decision-free and control-free, they acquire "learned helplessness," a condition which may lead to reactive depression and may be related to physical decline. Learned helplessness may also lead to indirect self-destructive behavior, which is often manifested in behaviors such as alcoholism, obesity, withdrawal from a social environment, disregard for or abuse of one's health, and suicide.

022   **Miller, Douglas K., & Kaiser, Fran E. (February, 1993). Assessment of the older woman.** *Clinics in Geriatric Medicine,* **9(1), 1-32.**

The author discusses the issue of general health assessment for elderly women (ages 60 and over). Sensory function, continence, nutrition, risk of falls, upper extremity function, strength, cognitive status, psychological status, bone integrity, sexual function, alcohol use and abuse, medication use, economic status, living status, and home environment are all important areas for assessment that may present problems for elderly women. The author gives recommendations for a complete, yearly screening starting at age 60, and suggests that adequate screening can improve diagnosis, intervention, and treatment outcomes in elderly women.

023   National Committee for Injury Prevention and Control. (1989). *Injury prevention: Meeting the Challenge.* New York: Oxford University Press.

This report describes the process and substance of injury prevention, explaining how to plan, implement, and interpret data from injury prevention programs. Several specific injury topics are discussed: traffic injuries, residential injuries, recreational injuries, occupational injuries, violence and injury, assaultive injuries, child abuse, domestic violence, elder abuse, rape and sexual assault, suicide, and firearm injuries. For each of these topics, the authors include statistical data concerning the magnitude of the injury, the cost, at-risk groups and risk factors, currently used interventions, and the committee's recommendations for future research and interventions.

024   National Safety Council. (1992). *Accident facts, 1992 edition.* Itasca, IL: National Safety Council.

This book has tables, charts, and graphs showing the ways people died from accidents in 1991. During this year, the number of accidental deaths (88,000) was the lowest reported in 70 years. Most types of accidental deaths decreased, except firearm injuries (+8%) and poisoning (+2%). The book classifies accidents by type, age, state, month, and other variables. Major classifications include all accidents, work accidents, occupational health, motor vehicle accidents, public accidents, home accidents, farm resident accidents, and environmental health. Information on the types and numbers of accidental deaths are reported in this publication. Deaths and death rates are presented by age and gender.

025   National Safety Council. (1993). *Accident facts, 1993 edition.* Itasca, IL: National Safety Council.

This book contains statistics on deaths caused by accidents in 1992 by age, state, type, and other variables. The total number of accidental deaths (83,000) was the lowest reported since 1922. Motor vehicle accidents were responsible for nearly 50% of all accidental deaths. The authors identify motor vehicle accidents (a broad category including pedestrian accidents) as the most common cause of accidental death for older Americans.

026 National Safety Council. (1994). *Accident facts, 1994 edition.* Itasca, IL: National Safety Council.

This book contains statistics on deaths caused by unintentional injuries in 1993 by age, state, type, and other variables. During this year, the number of unintentional injury deaths and the population death rate increased for the first time in five years. Motor vehicle injury deaths increased 3%, home injury deaths increased 7%, and public injury deaths increased 8%. Adults ages 65 and over had a higher death rate than the general population.

027 *Pep up your life: A fitness book for seniors.* (undated). Washington, DC: American Association of Retired Persons.

This book is a practical guide on exercise for the elderly that gives advice on nutrition, sleep and rest, and safe ways for the elderly to exercise. The program described in this book is organized by different levels of flexibility, strength, and endurance to allow gradual progress using exercises suitable for each individual's fitness level. Some of the exercises illustrated in the book may also be used by people in wheelchairs.

028 Rice, Dorothy P., MacKenzie, Ellen J., & Associates. (1989). *Cost of injury in the United States: A report to Congress.* San Francisco, CA: Institute for Health & Aging, University of California and Injury Prevention Center, The Johns Hopkins University.

This book evaluates the impact of injury on individuals, government programs, and society at large, including both the economic cost and the effects of injury. The authors use comprehensive data on incidence, cause, severity, lifetime cost, and life year and productivity losses from leading causes injury to provide the foundation for recommendations concerning future injury prevention research and funding. The leading causes of injury include motor vehicle, falls, firearms, poisonings, fires and burns, drownings and near-drownings.

029 Robertson, Leon S. (1992). *Injury Epidemiology.* New York: Oxford University Press.

The author discusses epidemiological methods for studying injuries and evaluating prevention interventions, suggesting that the nature of research questions and research methods may be the key to conducting accurate epidemiology research. Injury prevention programs can be improved with the help of relatively simple descriptive studies, but some necessary elements can only be evaluated by more sophisticated analysis. The book describes methods of injury surveillance, epidemiological analysis, determining behavioral factors and interventions, researching laws concerning behavior, and other issues related to injury epidemiology and data analysis.

030   Rockett, Ian R. H., & Smith, Gordon S. (October, 1989). Homicide, suicide, motor vehicle crash, and fall mortality: United States' experience in comparative perspective. *American Journal of Public Health, 79*(10), 1396-1401.

The authors compared data on motor vehicle crash, fall, suicide, and homicide mortality in the United States with similar data from France, Japan, West Germany, and the United Kingdom. Motor vehicle crashes were the predominant cause of injury death in the United States, and similar rates were shown in the other countries studied except Japan. Fall-related deaths were most common among the elderly; however, the authors suggest that these figures show underreporting due to other complications that may cloud the actual cause of death. The rate of fall-related deaths is higher in France and West Germany than in the United States. The elderly also showed the greatest rates of suicide, although rates between countries varied by age and gender. Although homicide is responsible for fewer deaths than motor vehicle crashes or suicide, the rate for the United States is much higher than for the other countries studied. This is largely due to the number of handgun-related homicides in the United States, and the strict handgun regulations in the comparison countries. The authors suggest that further research in the injury rate differences between countries may help identify the actual causes and risk factors associated with increased risk of injury deaths.

031   Roybal, Charlotte. (1993). *New Mexico, 1993: Injury.* Santa Fe, NM: New Mexico Department of Health.

This publication discusses injury categories as they relate to different age groups in New Mexico, and gives prevention techniques for each. Topics include falls, motor vehicle crashes, poisoning, and drowning, and intentional injuries like homicide, assault, abuse, and suicide, traumatic brain and spinal cord injuries, problem use of alcohol, and firearm injuries. Each topic is described with current statistical data on prevalence, risk factors, and costs incurred for each type of injury. The author also gives prevention recommendations for each type of injury.

032 Schappert, Susan M. (August 18, 1994). National ambulatory medical care survey: 1992 summary. *Advance Data, 253,* 1-20.

In 1992, the United States population made an average of three visits per person to an office-based physician. More than half of these visits were to a physician who specialized in general or family practice, internal medicine, or pediatrics. About 9% of visits were to an obstetrician or gynecologist. Other specialties included ophthalmology, orthopedic surgery, dermatology, general surgery, otolaryngology, psychiatry, urological surgery, cardiovascular diseases, and neurology. All other specialists made up 7.9% of the visits. Approximately 8.6% of all visits were related to an injury. Males made 56.7% of injury-related visits. The survey showed that 10.3% of those who visited a doctor smoked cigarettes. People between ages 65 and 74 made 11.9% of the visits and people over 75 accounted for an additional 10.1%. Of all of the injury-related visits, people between ages 65 and 74 made 5.5% of office visits, with people ages 75 and over accounting for an additional 4.5%. Counseling for alcohol abuse was ordered or provided in 3,161,000 visits, with males receiving alcohol counseling twice as often as females. The most common diagnoses made by doctors was hypertension, followed by pregnancy, upper respiratory infection, otitis media, chronic sinusitis, and diabetes. Among people ages 65 and over, the leading medical condition was hypertension, hypercholesterolemia, obesity, and depression. Females were more likely to be obese and depressed than males.

033 Schwarz, Donald F., Grisso, Jeane Ann, Miles, Carolyn G., Holmes, John H., Wishner, Amy R., & Sutton, Rudolph L. (March 9, 1994). A longitudinal study of injury morbidity in an African-American population. *Journal of the American Medical Association, 271*(10), 755-760.

This study used data from 11 hospital emergency departments in Philadelphia, Pennsylvania to examine the patterns of injury morbidity and mortality in an African American population. A total of 42,260 injury events were reported from 1987-1990, of which 2,796 resulted in admission to the hospital, and 403 resulted in death. In 1987, falls were the most frequent cause of injury, but by 1989, interpersonal intentional injuries were more common than falls. During the four years studied, firearm-related interpersonal intentional injuries went up 179%. Of males ages 20 to 29, 94.3% visited the emergency room at least once because of an injury, and 40.9% received treatment for one or more interpersonal intentional injuries. The authors suggest that injury prevention in urban populations should target interpersonal intentional injuries, and that injury prevention efforts on a general population level may be more effective than efforts targeted to smaller groups.

034   *Staying well: Health promotion programs for older persons.* **(1994). Washington, DC: American Association of Retired Persons.**

This book describes the many resources and types of health promotion programs available for use among the elderly. The authors discuss how to decide what kind of program to use, and give practical ways to implement the program. Several health promotion programs are listed by area of emphasis, and described according to any relevant statistical information, what activities are involved, personnel and material needs, costs, how to begin, and additional resources to help with the program.

035   **Steffl, Bernita M. (Ed.) (1984).** *The Handbook of Gerontological Nursing.* **New York: Van Nostrand Reinhold Company.**

This book is a guide for gerontological nurses. In addition to general gerontology and nursing principles, the book describes methods of health assessment, clinical conditions common among the elderly, and the rehabilitation needs of elderly patients. Individual chapters are devoted to special issues related to caring for older adults: nutrition, drugs, ethnic and cultural issues, sexuality, pressure ulcers, long term care, and gerontological nursing research. A chapter on unintentional injury and immobility describes the most common injuries among the elderly (falls, foot problems, dental and oral problems, hypothermia, hyperthermia, choking, elder abuse, and fires) and gives practical solutions to prevent and treat these types of injuries.

036   **Tanner, Elizabeth K. Wilhide. (December, 1991). Assessment of a health-promotive lifestyle.** *Nursing Clinics of North America,* **26(4), 845-854.**

The author describes a method that nurses may use to assess a patient's need for health promotion intervention. This assessment has four parts: 1. health history and physical assessment, which includes measures of general physical health as well as sexual and family planning histories; 2. assessment of health-promoting behaviors, which includes evaluating the patient's nutrition, physical activity, and stress management; 3. assessment of health-protecting behaviors, which includes preventing the use of tobacco and abuse of alcohol or other substances as well as avoiding environmental hazards and injury; and 4. evaluating resources, which include the patient's psychological health, spiritual dimension, and social lifestyle. The author suggests that the information gained by a complete assessment will help the nurse and the patient make informed decisions to improve the quality of life and health of the patient.

037   Teret, Stephen P., & Jacobs, Michael. (1989). Prevention and torts: The role of litigation in injury control. *Law, Medicine & Health Care, 17*(1), 17-22.

This article describes the legal aspects of injury control, especially those concerning product liability. Unfortunately, the product liability lawsuits (torts) that receive the most attention are not those which serve this purpose, and the negative publicity has led some to seek stricter regulation of these lawsuits. The authors suggest that if manufacturers and retailers are held financially responsible for unsafe products, there will be an incentive for them to participate in injury prevention. This concept may also applied to medical malpractice.

038   Teutsch, Steven M. (March 27, 1992). A framework for assessing the effectiveness of disease and injury prevention. *Morbidity and Mortality Weekly Report, 41*(RR-3), 1-12.

This report gives an overview of a method used to evaluate disease and injury prevention programs. Any assessment of prevention programs should include identifying the effectiveness of the strategies used, determining the potential and practical consequences of those strategies, evaluating the economic impact of the program, determining the best way to implement the program, and evaluating the impact of the program.

039   U. S. Consumer Product Safety Commission. (1986). *Safety for older consumers: Home safety checklist*. Washington, DC: U. S. Consumer Product Safety Commission.

This booklet is a checklist for fire and other safety hazards in the home directed at older adults. Recommendations include replacing frayed electrical cords, regularly testing smoke detectors, installing non-skid surfaces and grab bars in bathrooms, and throwing out old medications. The authors suggest that the checklist can be used as a resource for future reference and for periodic home safety checks.

040   U. S. Preventive Services Task Force. (1990). **Counseling to prevent household and environmental injuries.** *American Family Physician, 42*(1), 135-142.

This article discusses the effectiveness of physician counseling on the prevention of injuries. the authors suggest, even though there is no conclusive evidence of effectiveness, that physicians should counsel their patients about injury prevention because of the cost and suffering burden that injuries produce. Alcohol and drug use is a proven risk factor for injuries, so physicians should counsel their patients to avoid high-risk activities while intoxicated. The incidence of injuries such as falls, bicycle injuries, drowning, fires and burns, poisoning, and firearm injuries may also be reduced as a result of physician counseling, especially with patients in high-risk groups.

041   **Viano, David C. (July-August, 1990). A blueprint for injury control in the United States.** *Public Health Reports, 105*(4), 329-333.

The author describes a National Academy of Sciences' review of a Centers for Disease Control injury control program, which applauded the success of the program and made several recommendations for future programs. These recommendations include organizing the effort into an institute, seeking appropriate funding for further research, balancing the five areas of injury control (epidemiology, prevention, biomechanics, acute care, and rehabilitation), continuing the evaluation of existing programs, and establishing an advisory council to create a blueprint for future injury control programs based on the Centers for Disease Control model.

042   **Wallace, Robert B., & Woolson, Robert F. (Eds.). (1992).** *The epidemiologic study of the elderly.* **New York: Oxford University Press.**

This book is a review of the issues related to investigating the health problems of the elderly as a population. Before studying the elderly as a group, researchers should have an understanding of basic gerontology, as well as a knowledge of the complications of illness and the methodology of prevention for this population. The authors discuss the ethical and methodological aspects of surveying and assessing the elderly using existing studies to illustrate the difficult nature of research among this population.

043 Waller, Julian A. (February, 1987). Injury as disease. *Accident Analysis and Prevention, 19*(1), 13-20.

The author discusses the disease concept of injury as it relates to prevention measures, explaining the theory's advantages and limitations, and applying the theory to alcohol-related injuries. Viewing injury as a disease emphasizes the external sources of energy causing the injury, rather than the victim's behavior. For instance, disease-based methods of preventing motor vehicle crashes would be improvements in roads and motor vehicles that would decrease the environmental risk of crashing and subsequent injury. Traditional prevention methods would include education for drivers that emphasized safe driving practices. The author suggests that neither theory of prevention can be used exclusively; instead, prevention interventions should be selected based on which methods are not only theoretically sound, but are also effective and practical. Viewing injury as a disease can allow public health professionals the option to apply environmental interventions that may be more effective and less costly to society than behavioral methods. The author illustrates his argument by discussing the relationship of alcohol to injury, and the ways in which both behavioral and environmental interventions may be applied to prevent alcohol-related injuries and deaths.

044 Waller, Julian A. (1985). *Injury control: A guide to the causes and prevention of trauma.* Lexington, MA: D.C. Heath and Company.

This book describes the three phases of injury (pre-injury, injury, and post-injury) and the pathways of injury: kinetic energy, thermal energy, chemical energy, electrical energy, and ionizing radiation. The book also describes specific injury events such as motor vehicle, bicycle, and pedestrian events; injuries at home; burns; scalds; hypothermia; falls, and poisoning. Construction features and tools for living such as stairs, doors, windows, tubs and showers, furnishings, appliances, and housewares can play a part in injury events. The book also describes high-risk populations such as children, youths, and the elderly, as well as several injury settings: hospitals, nursing homes, the workplace, and recreational areas.

2

Alcohol and Problem Use

The issue of problem use of alcohol has two major dimensions. First there are those elderly people who are dependent on alcohol or who drink heavily, often referred to in the literature as alcoholics. The other dimension is the relationship of moderate use of alcohol and the injuries to which the elderly are prone such as falls, medication reactions, and driving accidents. Alcohol use is also associated with nearly every other classification of injury addressed in this book. This chapter includes articles and books dealing with prevalence issues, costs, risk factors, hazards, and prevention related to both alcoholism and moderate use of alcohol. Articles related to the role of alcohol as risk factors for specific injuries such as falls, drowning, motor vehicle accidents, and others are included in the chapters on those topics. Information related to the use of screening instruments used to identify problem use of alcohol is also included. Information specifically related to treatment of alcoholism is not included unless the article includes a discussion of treatment concerns as part of a broader approach to the subject.

045   Abrams, Robert C., & Alexopoulos, George S. (1987). Substance abuse in the elderly: Alcohol and prescription drugs. *Hospital and Community Psychiatry, 38*(12), 1285-1287.

This literature review discusses recent research on elderly alcoholism and abuse or misuse of prescription drugs. The authors recommend that substance abuse, misuse, and dependence be considered in the evaluation of every geriatric patient, including those residing in nursing homes. They also recommend considering hospitalization for elderly people who become dependent on alcohol or prescription drugs.

046   **Adams, Wendy L., Garry, Philip J., Rhyne, Robert, Hunt, William C., & Goodwin, James S. (March, 1990). Alcohol intake in the healthy elderly. Changes with age in a cross-sectional and longitudinal study. *Journal of the American Geriatrics Society, 38*(3), 211-216.**

The authors conducted both cross-sectional and longitudinal analyses of alcohol use in 270 healthy elderly persons over a seven-year period (1980 to 1987). Alcohol consumption was assessed by three-day diet records. One hundred sixty-five subjects (61.1%) remained in the study until 1987; 143 (53%) completed diet records for every year. Longitudinal analysis showed a statistically significant decline in the percent of subjects consuming any alcohol over time. A cross-sectional analysis of the 1980 data revealed a similar decline in the percentage drinkers with increasing age. Mean alcohol intake for those who continued to drink did not change over time except among heavy drinkers who consumed greater than 30 grams per day in 1980. These subjects showed a significant decline in mean alcohol intake. In this population the decline in the percentage of drinkers as they aged found in the cross-sectional analysis was confirmed in longitudinal analyses, suggesting that this represented a true age-related decline rather than a cohort effect.

047   **Adams, Wendy L., Magruder-Habib, Kathryn, Trued, Sally, & Broome, Harry L. (December, 1992). Alcohol abuse in elderly emergency department patients. *Journal of the American Geriatrics Society, 40*(12), 1236-1240.**

This cross-sectional study assessed the prevalence of alcohol abuse in elderly emergency department (ED) patients, the prevalence of alcohol abuse for various categories of illness and injury among these patients, and the frequency of detection of elderly alcohol abusers by ED physicians. The subjects were 205 patients ages 65 and over who came to the ED of a 625-bed university hospital that serves a mixed urban and rural population during an eight-week period. Data were obtained from a structured interview, which included the CAGE questionnaire and other questions regarding alcohol use, ED records, and past medical records. The prevalence of lifetime alcohol abuse (CAGE positive or self-reported drinking problem) was 24%. The prevalence of current alcohol abuse (CAGE positive or self-reported drinking problem and alcohol use within the last year) was 14%. There was a particularly high prevalence (22%) among patients with gastrointestinal problems and a lower prevalence (7%) among those who presented with falls or other trauma. Physicians detected only 21% of the current alcohol abusers. The authors concluded that while alcohol abuse is a prevalent and important problem among elderly ED patients, it is not well detected by physicians in this setting. Alcohol abuse appears to be less common among elderly trauma patients than their younger counterparts, but is very common among patients with gastrointestinal problems.

048   Adams, Wendy L., Yuan, Zhong, Barboriak, Joseph J., & Rimm, Alfred A. (September 8, 1993). Alcohol related hospitalizations of elderly people: Prevalence and geographic variation in the United States. *Journal of the American Medical Association, 270*(10), 1222-1225.

The purpose of this cross-sectional study was to determine the prevalence, geographic variation, and charges to Medicare of alcohol-related hospitalizations for the elderly. All hospital inpatient Medicare Part A beneficiaries ages 65 and older were examined. The data revealed that alcohol was related in 54.7 per 10,000 population for men and 14.8 for women. In 1989, there were 33,039 alcohol-related cases at a cost of $233,543,500. There was considerable geographic variation. Prevalence ranged from 18.9 per 10,000 in Arkansas to 77.0 per 10,000 in Alaska. The authors conclude that alcohol-related hospitalizations among elderly people are about the same as for myocardial infarction.

049   Akers, Ronald L, La Greca, Anthony J., Cochran, John, & Sellers, Christine. (1989). Social learning theory and alcohol behavior among the elderly. *The Sociological Quarterly, 30*(4), 625-638.

This study extends the application of social learning theory to older adults' alcohol behavior. Data were gathered through face-to-face interviews of 1,410 people ages 60 and over living in New Jersey and Florida in either age homogeneous or age-integrated communities. Consumption frequency and quantity were assessed using a self-report measure of how often the subjects drank alcohol during the past 12 months. A social learning model of differential association, differential reinforcement, and definitions is supported by findings on elderly drinking behavior. In this sample, 38.2% reported no drinking; 21.4% reported daily drinking; 5.7% reported heavy drinking, and 0.7% reported excessive drinking. The authors concluded that drinking among the elderly is related to the norms and behavior of one's primary groups, one's own attitudes toward alcohol, and the balance of reinforcement for drinking.

050   Alexander, Francesca, & Duff, Robert W. (1988). Social interaction and alcohol use in retirement communities. *The Gerontologist, 28*(5), 632-636.

A study of 260 people living in retirement communities revealed that they were more likely to drink on a regular basis than elderly persons in the nation as a whole. Respondents included 21.5% abstainers and 46% regular drinkers as compared to 45% and 28% nationally. The authors suggest that this difference could be explained in two ways. First, it is possible that the residents of retirement communities are representative of a population that drinks more than another. This conclusion is based on findings indicating that elderly people with higher incomes and more education drink more than those with lower incomes and less education. In this case, the greater use of alcohol could be related to the financial and educational background of the "typical" retirement community resident. Second, the data in this article suggest that the social nature of retirement community life lends itself to more frequent social drinking. Some of the residents interviewed indicated that drinking was an integral part of social life in their community.

051   Atkinson, Roland M. (Ed.). (1984). *Alcohol and drug abuse in old age.* Washington, DC: American Psychiatric Press, Inc.

This book presents an overview of alcohol and drug abuse among the elderly with chapters by Roland Atkinson, Sheldon Zimberg, and other well-known writers in the field.

052   Atkinson, Roland M. (1987). Alcohol problems of the elderly. *Alcohol & Alcoholism, 22*(4), 415-417.

This essay postulates that neither gerontologists nor addictionologists tend to regard problem drinking by the elderly as a clinical phenomenon worthy of much concern. As a result there has been little development of clinical knowledge of the course, complications, treatment, and prevention of alcohol problems in the elderly. The author cites evidence from several studies that suggest that alcohol problems among the elderly constitute a moderate public health concern and that improved prevention, recognition and abatement is needed.

053 Barnea, Zipora, & Teichman, Meir. (1994). Substance misuse and abuse among the elderly: Implications for social work intervention. *Journal of Gerontological Social Work, 21(3-4)*, 133-149.

This article reviews the literature on the misuse and abuse of psychoactive substances among the elderly. Three main patterns of abuse for this age group are identified and analyzed: medications, alcohol, and illegal drugs. The article discusses the prevalence and incidence of substance abuse among the elderly, its predictors and correlates, its special dangers and effects on the elderly and their environment, and the roles that social workers should play in prevention and treatment.

054 Barnes, Grace M. (1979). Alcohol use among older persons: Findings from a western New York State general population survey. *Journal of the American Geriatrics Society, 27(6)*, 244-250.

This widely cited report on the drinking patterns of older persons is based upon a cross-sectional probability sample of 1,041 adults ages 18 and over living in Erie and Niagara Counties in Western New York State. The rates of drinking, heavy drinking, and alcohol-related problems were considerably lower among persons ages 60 and over than among those ages 50 to 59, or among those ages 18 to 49. Although heavy drinking was almost nonexistent among the elderly women, about a quarter of the men in the 60 to 69 age group were heavy drinkers. Previous reports concluding that the stresses of aging, such as widowhood and retirement, are associated with increased problem drinking were not confirmed in this study.

055 Bercsi, Stephen J., Brickner, Philip W., & Saha, Dhanonjoy C. (September, 1993). Alcohol use and abuse in the frail, home bound elderly: A clinical analysis of 103 persons. *Drug and Alcohol Dependence, 33(2)*, 139-150.

The authors studied alcohol use and abuse in 103 frail, homebound elderly individuals (mean age 80.63 years) cared for in a long-term home health care program from July 1991 to February 1992. Subjects completed the Mini-Mental Status Test, the CAGE, the SMAST, and answered additional questions regarding the use of tobacco, sedative/, and alcohol. Patients were classified into non-drinkers, past social drinkers, current social drinkers, and heavy drinkers (past and current). Heavy drinkers were those who consumed three or more drinks daily or drank twice or more daily. Non-drinkers were those who had consumed a minimal amount of alcohol in their lifetimes. Of the 103 subjects, 72 were women, 95 were white. The majority lived alone. There were 19 nondrinkers (18%), 43 past social drinkers (42%), 14 current social drinkers (13.5%), and 27 heavy drinkers (2 current and 25 past who were currently abstainers). All of the heavy drinking had started prior to age 45. Tobacco and sedative-hypnotics were associated with alcohol use and abuse. Sleep disturbance was more common in social drinkers. The authors concluded that a small percentage of their population actively uses or abuses alcohol (14% social, 2% heavy drinkers).

056   Beresford, Thomas P., Blow, Frederic C., & Brower, Kirk J. (September, 1990). Alcoholism in the elderly. *Comprehensive Therapy, 16*(9), 38-43.

This article discusses the diagnosis and treatment of elderly alcoholism or alcohol dependence. Diagnosis of alcoholism rests on four factors: tolerance to alcohol, withdrawal symptoms on cessation of alcohol use, loss of control of drinking behavior, and social decline. Elderly people, they point out, have a good prognosis for improvement once in treatment.

057   Bienenfeld, David. (August, 1987). Alcoholism in the elderly. *American Family Physician, 36*(2), 163-172.

This article reviews the unique factors of alcohol problems in elderly people, including drinking patterns, decreased tolerance of alcohol, drug interactions, and risks that increase with age. Because many methods of evaluation and treatment for younger alcoholics often do not apply to older patients, these factors must be considered. A moderate drinker may encounter serious health risks and problems as he or she ages, such as confusion, falls, emotional lability, and adverse drug interactions. These problems, if recognized by a physician, can be used to focus on the alcohol problem, and can lead to an effective treatment program.

058   Blazer, Dan, Crowell, Bradford A., & George, Linda K. (August, 1987). Alcohol abuse and dependence in the rural South. *Archives of General Psychiatry, 44,*(8), 736-740.

The authors studied rural–urban differences in the prevalence alcohol abuse or dependence from a community survey of 3,921 adults living in North Carolina. Analyses disclosed that current alcohol–related problems, as identified by the Diagnostic Interview Schedule, were more common in the rural area (4.2% vs. 2.6%). When the authors controlled for potential confounders, including age, sex, race, socioeconomic status, and the DIS–DSM–III diagnoses of major depression and antisocial personality disorder, the odds of alcohol abuse or dependence in the rural area remained significant for the "rural blacks." The authors concluded that factors leading to urban–rural differences in psychiatric disorders, such as current alcohol abuse or dependence, are more complex than can be explained by geographic boundaries alone.

059 **Blose, Irvin L. (January, 1978). The relationship of alcohol to aging and the elderly.** *Alcoholism: Clinical and Experimental Research, 2(1),* **17-21.**

The purpose of this literature research was to investigate the source of alcohol abuse among the elderly, the scope and nature of that abuse, and to examine the incidence and prevalence of the problem. Alcohol may be related to diminution of function in tissues and organ systems as well as individuals. Aging cells, systems, and people may respond differently to alcohol. The author concludes that the problem of alcohol abuse among people ages 65 and over, including those in nursing homes, is larger than had previously been estimated. He calls for attention to the problem by gerontologists and physicians.

060 **Blow, F. C., Brower, K. J., Schulenberg, J. E., Demo-Dananberg, L. M., Young, J. P., & Beresford, T. P. (1991).** *Michigan alcoholism screening test—Geriatric version (MAST-G): A new elderly-specific screening instrument.* **Ann Arbor, MI: University of Michigan.**

The MAST-G is the first elderly-specific alcoholism screening measure to be developed with items unique to older problem drinkers. This screening test consists of 24 questions in which alcoholism in the elderly can be detected. Because existing screening instruments had been shown to poorly identifying alcoholism among older adults, the authors developed a new screening instrument to address this clinical need. Items were developed based on a literature review of alcoholism among the elderly, a critique by a panel of alcoholism treatment professionals, and a focus group discussion by recovering older alcoholics. The 94 items of the initial instrument were tested on a heterogeneous sample of 840 older adults. The preliminary MAST-G was then reduced using a combination of item and factor analysis. The reduced instrument, consisting of 32 items, was refined using a stratified sample of 305 elderly subjects that included five groups: 1. those currently meeting criteria for alcohol dependence, but not in treatment; 2. those currently in treatment for alcoholism, 3. those with a previous history of alcoholism and currently in recovery, 4. social drinkers, and 5. abstainers. The diagnosis of alcohol dependence (DSM–III–R) was used as the validation standard. This process yielded a final version of 24 items. Psychometric properties of this new instrument are superior to other screening tests for identification of elderly alcoholics. The MAST-G has a sensitivity of 93.9%, specificity of 78.1%, positive predictive value of 87.2%, and negative predictive value of 88.9%. In addition, factor analysis identified five underlying symptom domains: Loss and loneliness, relaxation, dependence, loss of control with drinking, and rule–making.

061   Borgatta, Edgar F., Montgomery, Rhonda J. V., & Borgatta, Marie L. (September, 1982). Alcohol use and abuse, life crisis events, and the elderly. *Research on Aging, 4(3), 378–408.*

This retrospective study investigated alcohol abuse and the elderly. The authors point out the lack of consistent studies related to prevalence of problem use of alcohol. They state that the evidence strongly supports the idea that people drink less on average as they age. They reject the idea that there are two types of elderly alcoholics: early-onset, and late-onset. They also reject the idea the theory that there is an association between life stresses and late-life alcohol use. They conducted an analysis of data from the National Opinion Research Center (NORC) General Social Survey sample available for the years 1978 to 1980, dividing subjects into those ages 65 and over, ages 64 and under, and ages 45 and over. They found that there was a reduction of variance for age as well as a reduction in drinking. Females report drinking less than men, and people with higher education and with higher income report drinking more often. Church attenders and rural dwellers drink less. Whites drink more often than blacks. Smokers drink more than nonsmokers. The findings also do not support the theory that older people are less able to cope with stress and use drinking as an inappropriate coping behavior. The authors point out a number of flaws in many studies of alcohol use among the elderly. They stress that it is important to recognize that current procedures may be comparing alcoholics with medical problems to nonalcoholics in the general population.

062   Brennan, Penny L., Moos, Rudolf H., & Kim, Julia Y. (1993). Gender differences in the individual characteristics and life

contexts of late-middle-aged and older problem drinkers. *Addictions, 88,* 781-790.

This study focuses on gender differences in the individual characteristics and life contexts of late-life problem drinkers. The subjects were 704 people (509 men, 195 women) who were between ages 55 and 65 (mean age 61 years) with a current drinking problem. Measures assessed substance abuse and depression, help-seeking efforts, and life stressors and social resources. They also assessed alcohol consumption, use of psychoactive drugs, depression, and age of onset. Results showed a number of gender differences. Women consumed less alcohol, had fewer drinking problems, and reported more recent onset of drinking problems than did their male counterparts. They also used more psychoactive medications, were more depressed, and were less likely to seek alcohol treatment. Consistent with a gender role perspective on alcohol abuse, problem-drinking women had more family-related and fewer financial stressors than did problem-drinking men. The women reported more support from children, extended family members, and friends than did problem-drinking men. Women who continued to have drinking problems over a one-year interval reported some short-term benefits at follow-up, including reduced spouse stressors. Women who were not drinking at follow-up experienced less spouse support, and more family-related stressors and depression than did remitted men. They also lost support from extended family members over the one-year interval. The results suggest a need for screening and treatment efforts tailored more closely to the life circumstances of women with drinking problems in late life.

063 Brower, Kirk J., Mudd, Sharon, Blow, Frederic C., Young, James P., & Hill, Elizabeth M. (February, 1994). Severity and treatment of alcohol withdrawal in elderly versus younger patients. *Alcoholism, Clinical and Experimental Research,* 18(1), 196-201.

The purpose of this study was to determine whether elderly alcoholics experienced a more severe course of withdrawal that younger alcoholics. The authors conducted a retrospective chart review of 48 older (mean age 60 years) and 36 younger (mean age 30 years) patients in a residential center being treated for alcohol withdrawal. Overall, elderly alcoholics experienced significantly more withdrawal symptoms for a longer time than younger alcoholics. None of the patients had seizures during the withdrawal. The older group was much more likely to suffer from cognitive impairment, weakness, and high blood pressure. This study provides a detailed description of the characteristics of the population of elderly alcoholic studied.

064   **Brown, Bradford B. (1982). Professionals' perceptions of drug and alcohol abuse among the elderly.** *The Gerontologist,* **22(6), 519-524.**

The author interviewed the chief administrators in 30 agencies in one midwestern county selected to form a representative sample of the professional services that deal with older people. The agencies were divided into three groups: drug abuse agencies, health care facilities, and housing and social services. The administrators identified 20 characteristics that they felt precipitated drug and alcohol abuse among the elderly. Four were mention by 25% of more of the sample: loss of productive social roles or functions, loneliness, acquiring a drinking habit earlier in life, and the absence of supportive social relationships. Perceptions of what caused drug and alcohol abuse among older people differed somewhat according to the type of services an agency offered or its approach to older abusers. Practitioners appeared to be concerned about the problem in older persons. One-third thought it was a minor problem, 25% thought it was a serious problem. Health care professionals expressed a relatively low level of concern. Education was recommended as an important community response.

065   **Brown, Bradford B., & Chiang, Chi-Pang. (1983-84). Drug and alcohol abuse among the elderly: Is being alone the key?** *International Journal of Aging and Human Development,* **18(1), 1-12.**

This study compared the social support relationships of older persons in treatment for drug or alcohol abuse to relationships among both older abusers not in treatment and nonabusers in the community at large. The sample consisted of 21 older people currently receiving professional help for drug or alcohol related problems, 153 older adults receiving some health or social services, but not for substance abuse, and 65 individuals residing in public housing. Each respondent participated in a structured interview. Analyses suggested that age and gender affect the likelihood of receiving treatment more than the likelihood of being an abuser. Age and gender were negatively associated with substance abuse. A higher number of abusers than nonabusers were currently separated or divorced. Those in treatment, however, were more likely to be living with someone else. The authors conclude that drug and alcohol abuse is an extensive problem among the elderly (ages 55 and over). In their sample, 14% of housing residents and social service clients were classified as abusers. They also conclude that older people n drug-abuse treatment programs are not necessarily representative of older substance abusers as a whole. They also believe that alcohol-abuse did not appear to be related to age, gender, race, or education variables found to be associated in other studies.

066   Buchsbaum, David G., Buchanan, Robin G., Welsh, Josephine, Centor, Robert M., & Schnoll, Sidney H. (July, 1992). Screening for drinking disorders in the elderly using the CAGE questionnaire. *Journal of the American Geriatrics Society, 40(7),* 662-665.

The purpose of this study was to assess the effectiveness of the CAGE questionnaire in identifying elderly outpatients with drinking problems. A cross-sectional design, with the alcohol module of the Diagnostic Interview Schedule as the criterion standard, was used in the outpatient medical practice of an urban university teaching hospital. The subjects were 323 patients who were 60 and older. Data were collected to assess the CAGE's sensitivity, specificity, receiver operating characteristics (ROC) curve and positive predictive value for CAGE scores of 0 to 4 for patients ages 60 and over. Researchers found that 33% of the sample met study criteria for a history of drinking problems, including 63% of the male patients and 22% of the female patients. The sensitivity and specificity for a cut-off score of one for all patients was 86% and 78%, respectively, and 70% and 91% for a cut-off of two. The calculation of the area under the ROC curve was 0.86, and the positive predictive value of CAGE scores of 0 to 4 were 33%, 66%, 79%, 82%, and 94%, respectively. The predictive value for any score was higher in males than females, reflecting the higher prevalence of problems in the male population. Buchsbaum and his colleagues concluded that the CAGE can effectively discriminate elderly patients with a history of drinking problems from those without such a history. They strongly recommend screening elderly patients for the presence of drinking problems.

067   Chaikelson, June Steinberg, Arbuckle, Tannis Y., Lapidus, Steven, & Gold, Dolores Pushkar. (March, 1994). Measurement of lifetime alcohol consumption. *Journal of Studies on Alcohol,* 55(2), 133-140.

The purpose of the study was to develop a measure of lifetime alcohol use that would be appropriate for an elderly sample with an extended history of drinking, to assess its reliability and validity, and then to use the instrument to examine lifetime alcohol use from a longitudinal, retrospective perspective. The Concordia Lifetime Drinking Questionnaire (CLDQ) was assessed with a group of 328 Canadian men (mean age 69 years). The CLDQ includes quantity and frequency questions on current beverage-specific alcohol use and a series of questions about the start of alcohol use. Drinking was assessed on two occasions approximately 33 months apart. Forty-six wives responded to questions about their husband's drinking. The reliability coefficient for lifetime drinking was 0.78. Validity was tested by comparing each wife's rating of her husband's drinking at present and at time of marriage with information provided by their husbands; the correlations were 0.87 and 0.72, respectively. Moderate correlations were obtained between the MAST and the CLDQ. The CLDQ was judged to be a reliable and valid measure of lifetime drinking, appropriate for use with the elderly. The longitudinal lifetime drinking patterns appeared similar to those found in cross-sectional studies.

068   Cook, Brian L., Winokur, George, Garvey, Michael J., & Beach, Vickie. (January, 1991). Depression and previous alcoholism in the elderly. *British Journal of Psychiatry, 158*(1), 72-75.

The purpose of this study was to determine whether previous history of alcoholism significantly influenced treatment or response to treatment. The subjects were a group of male inpatients ages 55 and over who met Feighner criteria for non-bipolar depression. Among 58 subjects with complete follow-up information, the 16 who had a history of alcoholism had a presentation at index which differed from that of the non-alcoholics, and on follow-up they clearly had more chronic illness. The authors concluded that this elderly sample with alcoholism resembles "neurotic-reactive" depressives described in younger samples, and supports a past history of alcoholism as being a risk factor for chronicity of depression on follow-up in the elderly population.

069   Crossman, Lenard H. (Spring, 1984). Alcohol abuse in the elderly: Implications for educational and human service programming. *Journal of Alcohol and Drug Education, 29*(3), 31-34.

This review provides information about the alcoholism services available to the older American. Crossman points out the reasons why the elderly have been overlooked and underserved by the treatment and prevention services as 1. they are a poor risk and resources can be better allocated elsewhere, 2. alcoholism is difficult to diagnose in the elderly population; 3. diagnostic criteria tend to exclude older adults. Older people, however, are as much an at-risk population as any other group. Treatment programs need to address the needs of problem drinkers other than alcoholics. Treatment programs need to be opened up to the elderly. The author concludes that programs for the elderly need to be given a higher priority.

070   Curtis, J. Randall, Geller, Gail, Stokes, Emma J., Levine, David M., & Moore, Richard D. (1989). Characteristics, diagnosis, and treatment of alcoholism in elderly patients. *Journal of the American Geriatrics Society, 37*(4), 310-316.

This article describes the diagnosis and the misdiagnosis of alcoholism in elderly patients. During a three-month period, new admissions to The Johns Hopkins Hospital were screened for alcoholism with both the CAGE questions and the SMAST. Of those ages 59 and under, 27% were positively identified by the screening, and 21% of the patients ages 60 and over were similarly identified. Of the younger group, 60% of the positively-screened group were correctly identified by the hospital. Only 37% of the elderly positive group were so identified, and even when the problem was correctly diagnosed, the elderly group were less likely to have treatment recommended to them, and further, that the treatment recommended was less likely to be initiated by the hospital. The authors conclude that physicians have not been trained to detect and treat elderly problem drinkers.

071   Cyr, Michele G., & Wartman, Steven A. (1988). The effectiveness of routine screening questions in the detection of alcoholism. *Journal of the American Medical Association, 259*(1), 51-54.

This study assessed the prevalence of alcoholism in an ambulatory medical clinic and the effectiveness of screening questions for alcoholism. The 232 subjects (ages 18 to 79) were interviewed using a questionnaire that included the Michigan Alcoholism Screening Test (MAST). Based on MAST scores, 47 (20.3%) of the subjects were identified as alcoholics. Sensitivities and specificities for alcohol–use questions were calculated using the MAST diagnosis of alcoholism. The questions "How much do you drink?" and "How often do you drink?" yielded low sensitivities of 34.0% and 46.8%, respectively. The question "Have you ever had a drinking problem?" considered alone had a high sensitivity of 70.2%. When combined with "When was your last drink?" this question had a sensitivity of 91.5%. The authors recommend the routine incorporation of these last two questions into the medical history in light of the high prevalence of alcoholism in this outpatient population. Results also showed a significant relationship between employment status, smoking, and family history of alcoholism. Alcoholics were more likely to be unemployed, smokers, and have a family history of alcoholism. Alcoholics and nonalcoholics did not differ on medical history, education, diet, exercise, or type of alcohol consumed.

072   Dufour, Mary C., Archer, Loran, & Gordis, Enoch. (February, 1992). Alcohol and the elderly. *Clinics in Geriatric Medicine, 8*(1), 127-141.

This comprehensive article discusses several questions related to the use of alcohol by elderly people. The authors investigate the benefits and problems related to the use of alcohol in moderate as well as abusive amounts. Moderate drinking for older people is defined as "no more than one drink per day." They explain age differences related to the effects of alcohol. The primary difference is due to diminishing lean body mass and increasing adipose tissue that accompanies aging causing the volume of total body water to decrease and thus produce a higher blood alcohol concentration. They also discuss the effects of alcohol on energy and morale noting that alcohol provides both caloric and "psychic energy." They point out that people using alcohol may decrease their food consumption, change their eating habits, and have less money for food. Malnutrition is a well-known complication of chronic alcoholism but not related to moderate use. They also discuss the effects of alcohol on cognitive function and conclude that for elderly people these effects are mostly negative. Insomnia is a common complaint of older people and alcohol with its sedative, hypnotic properties is often thought to be beneficial in producing sleep. They point out that while it initially promotes sleep it causes disturbances in sleep patterns that may create more problems than it solved. Research seems to support some beneficial effects of alcohol on appetite and digestion if taken in small amounts before meals. While heavy alcohol consumption is linked to increased risk of death from heart disease, moderate levels of consumption are often promoted as beneficial to the heart. Little research has been done, however, with older populations to either substantiate or deny that claim. Alcohol is also often used for relief of pain, particularly by arthritis sufferers. Pain relief, however, is temporary and there are better medications available for that purpose. Finally, the authors discuss the dangers of recommending moderate alcohol consumption to older people due to the variety of problems that could be triggered including preexisting alcohol problems, drug-alcohol interactions, and alcohol's potential for exacerbating cognitive impairment and dementias. The authors present the results of clinical studies on the therapeutic use of alcohol and conclude that for most older people, particularly those who are frail and living alone that great caution should be urged in encouraging alcohol consumption due to the risks of drug interaction and increased chance of falls due to impaired balance.

073 **Dunham, Roger G. (April-June, 1981). Aging and changing patterns of alcohol use.** *Journal of Psychoactive Drugs, 13*(2), 143-151.

The author investigated types of elderly alcoholic and different drinking patterns. Data were drawn from interviews with 310 subjects ages 60 and over living in government-funded, low-income housing for elderly people in Dade County, Florida; 73% were ages 70 and over using a self-reported retrospective measure of life-drinking patterns. Of the 360 people identified, 14% refused to be interviewed. Of the 310 people interviewed, 68% were life-long abstainers. Only 100 (32%) reported some drinking during their lifetimes. The high abstinence rate was explained by 67% female; a prohibition-era cohort. The sample consisted of 46% Anglo; 40% Latin; and 14% Black. Seven patterns of usage were identified: 1. life-long abstainers; 2. rise-and fall pattern (N=21, 25%); 3. rise-and-sustained pattern (N=24; 28%); 4. light throughout life pattern (N=18, 21%); 5. light with a late rise pattern (N=6, 7%); 6. late starters (N=9, 11%); and 7. highly variable patterns (N=7, 8%). Considerable movement in and out of the five categories of drinkers was observed during the respondents' lifetime. The most frequent reason for a decrease was because of a specific health problem. Females were more likely to be abstainers than males; married and widowed were the most likely to be abstainers. Latins were most likely to be abstainers; blacks were the least likely. Of the religious affiliations named, Catholics were most likely to be abstainers; respondents with no religious affiliation were the least likely to be abstainers. Level of education did not affect the results in this sample.

074   **Dunne, Francis J. (1994). Misuse of alcohol or drugs by elderly people.** *British Medical Journal, 308*(6929), 608-609.

This review article examines the problem of alcohol and/or drug misuse among elderly people. It is estimated that between 5% and 12% of men and 1% to 2% of women in their 60s are problem drinkers. A study of elderly men and women also reported that nearly one-fifth of both sexes who drank regularly exceeded the recommended limits. Because elderly people are more susceptible to the toxic effects of alcohol and at a higher risk for drug interactions, the author suggests that physicians should routinely obtain drug and alcohol use histories from elderly patients. Screening instruments appropriate for this age group are also needed. Treatment of elderly persons with alcohol or drug problems should be matched to the individual's particular needs.

075   **Dupree, Larry W., Broskowski, Helen, & Schonfeld, Lawrence. (Spring, 1984). Alcohol abuse in the elderly: Implications for educational and human service programming.** *The Gerontologist, 24*(5), 510-516.

This study assessed the effectiveness of the Gerontology Alcohol Project, a self management treatment program for adult-onset alcohol abusers. Results indicated a marked success for those completing the treatment program, including an improved social support network.

076   **Felson, David T., Kiel, Douglas P., Anderson, Jennifer J, & Kamel, William B. (November, 1988). Alcohol consumption and hip fractures: The Framingham Study.** *American Journal of Epidemiology, 128*(5), 1102-1110.

This study investigated the relationship between alcohol consumption and hip fracture in the Framingham Heart Study cohort, a population that has been studied longitudinally since the 1950s. Subjects had been asked about their alcohol consumption at eight different times. Data were also collected about hip fractures sustained by the subjects. For analysis, current alcohol intake was divided into three categories: light, moderate, and heavy. The heavy intake category (seven or more ounces per week) included 10% of the women and 25% of the men. Of the 217 hip fractures that occurred in the cohort, 174 occurred among women and 43 among men. Most fractures occurred in subjects ages 75 and over.

Data analysis showed that current heavy alcohol consumption increases the risk of hip fracture. Risk is increased substantially in those ages 65 and under. Even moderate alcohol intake significantly increased the risk of hip fracture in women ages 65 and under. The investigators concluded that the increased risk of fractures by alcoholics was attributable not only to increased risk of falling and motor vehicle accidents but also because of low bone density. They also suspected underreporting of alcohol intake by older women. This article provides considerable additional information about patterns of alcohol consumption.

077   Forster, Lorna Earl, Pollow, Rachel, & Stoller, Eleanor Palo. (1993). Alcohol use and potential risk for alcohol-related adverse drug reactions among community-based elderly. *Journal of Community Health, 18*(4), 225-239.

This paper documents the frequency of alcohol consumption and concurrent use of alcohol and medications in a random sample of elderly community dwellers, develops a profile of older people likely to use alcohol, and explores the extent to which they are at risk due to concurrent use of prescription and over-the-counter medications. The authors selected a sample of 667 people ages 65 and over from a four-county, nonmetropolitan area in northeast New York State, (mean age 74.1 years, SD=6.6). Respondents were asked about their alcohol consumption and use of medications. The majority of respondents (57%) reported using alcohol; 29.5% rarely; 16.3% sometimes; and 11.3% regularly. About 25% were potentially at risk for alcohol related adverse drug reactions (ADR) and 15% were at risk for multiple ADR. The most common risk was from the use of OTC pain medications and alcohol (19%). Sex, educational attainment, and religious affiliation were significantly related to risk for alcohol-related ADR. The author point out that beneficial effects of moderate use of alcohol may be outweighed by the potential for alcohol-related adverse reactions to medications.

078   Freund, Gerhard. (Spring, 1984). Current research directions on alcohol problems and aging. *Alcohol Health and Research World, 8*(5), 12-15.

This article discusses sequelae of aging including degeneration, diseases, and death. The author explains biological mechanisms and social influences related to consequences and causes of alcohol use and research related to the effects of alcohol on cognitive function. The author concludes that aging causes the decline of many tissues and functions, increased susceptibility to various diseases that are also encountered in younger persons, and eventually death. Alcohol molecules change tissues, organs, personal, and eventually social behavior. It is to be expected that chronic alcohol consumption may influence all three types of the sequelae of aging. At the present time, however, very little is known about the relationships between aging and alcohol at any level of biological organization.

079   Freund, Gerhard. (Winter, 1982). The interaction of chronic alcohol consumption and aging on brain structure and function. *Alcoholism, Clinical and Experimental Research, 6*(1), 13-21.

This article is a review of the literature on biological aging and alcohol abuse. Freund discusses alcohol and thiamin deficiency and alcohol and the aging central nervous system. He points out that cognitive performance declines moderately with normal aging and severely with pathological aging and that intellectual impairment is also associated with prolonged alcohol consumption. Freund concludes from the human and animal data he reviewed that chronic ethanol consumption appears to increase some behavioral deficits caused by aging. What the exact interrelationships are at the molecular basis for the behavioral changes is not yet clear.

080   Fuller, Richard K., & Gordis, Enoch. (August 17, 1994). Refining the treatment of alcohol withdrawal. *Journal of the American Medical Association, 272*(7), 557-558.

There are different drugs available to treat alcohol withdrawal. Physicians may be confused as to which one and which dosage regimen should be used as first-line therapy. Clonidine is effective for treatment of alcohol withdrawal symptoms but is not recommended as first-line therapy because it does not prevent seizures. Despite the availability of other drugs, benzodiazepines remain the preferred pharmacologic agents for treatment of acute alcohol withdrawal. Benzodiazepines have been shown to be effective for treating alcohol withdrawal.

081   Gomberg, Edith Lisansky. (1982). Special populations. In Edith Lisansky Gomberg, Helene Raskin White, & John A. Carpenter (Eds.), *Alcohol, science, and society revisited* (pp. 337-354). Ann Arbor: University of Michigan Press.

Gomberg discusses issues related to the elderly, and other special populations. She cites findings from her research indicating that the proportion of heavy drinkers decreases among both sexes at about age 50 and again for men around age 65. Also at about age 65 people a new group of problem drinkers seems to emerge. People who have abused alcohol throughout life are referred to as "survivors" and new problem drinkers are "reactives." She points out that since older people tend to drink at home they are less visible, particularly elderly men. The elderly alcoholic is most visible to family, friends and neighbors. She points out that many agencies and therapists are not responsive to the needs of older alcoholics even though there is evidence that they are very responsive to help. Gomberg also discusses issues related to adolescents, minorities, and women.

082   Gomberg, Edith S. Lisansky. (1988). Alcoholic women in treatment: The question of stigma and age. *Alcohol and Alcoholism, 23*(6), 507-514.

This study of 301 alcoholic women in treatment gathered information by a standardized life history interview was intended to gain information about the women's perception of social attitudes toward intoxication and problem drinking as compared to the women's own opinions on the subject. A matched group of non-alcoholic women were also interviewed. Both alcoholic women in treatment and a matched group of non-alcoholic women feel that social attitudes are more negative toward female intoxication and problem drinking than toward male intoxication and their drinking problems. Alcoholic women report significantly more negative attitudes, both social and personal, than do the non-alcoholic control women. Older alcoholic women are consistently harsher than younger ones in their judgments, both of social attitudes and in expression of their own opinions. When the total sample (alcoholic and non-alcoholic women) is compared in terms of positive family history versus negative family history, those with positive histories are more likely to agree with disapproving statements about women's problem drinking. Significantly more women with positive histories believe that social attitudes are more disapproving of women alcoholics than men, and they believe, to a significantly greater extent than those without such histories, that the effects of maternal alcoholism are worse than those of paternal alcoholism.

083   Goodwin, James S., Sanchez, Clare J., Thomas, Paula, Hunt, Curtis, Garry, Philip J., & Goodwin, Jean M. (February, 1987).

Alcohol intake in a healthy elderly population. *American Journal of Public Health, 77*(2), 173-177.

This study investigated drinking patterns of 270 healthy older people living independently in the community and the health consequences of alcohol use. The authors investigated the relationship between drinking patterns and age, gender, income, and education. Subjects recorded their diet for three days. Forty-eight percent of the sample recorded some alcohol intake, with 8% drinking 30 or more grams of alcohol daily. Alcoholic beverages were mostly wine and beer. Alcohol intake was positively associated with male gender, income, and amount of education and negatively associated with age. Alcohol intake was not associated with any changes in social or psychological status, but was positively associated with several measurements of cognitive status. These correlations were weak, however, and tended to disappear after controlling for income, education, gender, and age. Past alcohol intake was not associated with any indicators of present social, psychological, or cognitive functioning. The major finding of this study was that alcohol intake did not appear to have a negative effect on cognitive, psychological, or social status in this population.

084   Gorman, D. M., Werner, J. M., Jacobs, L. M., Duffy, S. W. (February, 1990). Evaluation of an alcohol education package for non-specialist health care and social workers. *British Journal of Addiction, 85*(2), 223-233.

This study evaluated the education package provided by the Drinking Problem Service in Cambridge to non-specialist agencies who have contact with problem drinkers. The design was a quasi-experimental non-equivalent control group design. The subjects' knowledge and attitudes were assessed using a modified version of the Alcohol and Alcohol Problems Perception Questionnaire (AAPPQ). One-month follow-up scores of the education teams were significantly higher than those of the controls, although the effect was stronger in the case of therapeutic attitudes than knowledge. There were also significant differences in improvement in attitude scores, with significant effects being observed in the general practice, medicine for the elderly and social work teams but not the accident and emergency. At six months, the level of fall-off in improvement varied.

085   Graham, Kathryn. (1986). Identifying and measuring alcohol abuse among the elderly: Serious problems with existing instrumentation. *Journal of Studies on Alcohol, 47(4),* 322-326.

This article points out the low rate of alcohol abuse among the elderly as compared to other age groups. Graham's view is that the elderly are underreported because existing instruments for identifying and measuring alcohol abuse are inappropriate for use with elderly populations because of differences between the young populations on which these measures were standardized and the elderly. Five domains used in measuring alcohol abuse 1. level of consumption, 2. alcohol-related social and legal problems, 3. alcohol-related health problems, 4. symptoms of drunkenness or dependence, and 5. self-recognition of the problem—and the extent to which these domains (as currently measured) apply to elderly populations are discussed. Graham recommends conducting studies to estimate reliability and validity of self-report among the elderly. Questions need to focus on problems that are experienced by women and men rather than exclusively men. Health problems related to alcohol abuse need to be identified. Importantly, the elderly need to be recognized as a heterogeneous group when it comes to alcohol abuse as well as non-abusive behavior.

086   Graham, Kathryn, Zeidman, Anne, Flower, Margaret C., Saunders, Sarah J., & White-Campbell, Marilyn. (1992). A typology of elderly persons with alcohol problems. *Alcoholism Treatment Quarterly, 9(3-4),* 79-96.

This study developed a typology of elderly alcohol abusers on the basis of 36 case studies conducted at an outreach addictions treatment program for the elderly. Three main types were defined: chronic alcohol abuser (abusive drinking primarily maintained by a life of habitual consumption and a lack of alternative activities), reactive problem drinker (alcohol abuse developed and maintained in response to a loss, such as ill health or death of a spouse), and problem drinkers whose drinking seemed to be interrelated with psychiatric or cognitive problems. The authors provide case descriptions to illustrate each type and the treatment implications of this typology are discussed.

087   Gross, Leonard. (1983). *How much is too much? The effects of social drinking.* New York: Random House.

This book brings attention to possible hazards of social drinking in the adult population. In Chapter 5, the author discusses potential benefits of moderate drinking including its psychotropic properties. He points out that the reason why abstainers compare favorably to moderate drinkers may be due to the reasons why the people are abstaining. He points out areas where alcohol, especially heavy use, threatens health, particularly its relationship to cirrhosis, cancer and hypertension. A second major issue is the relationship between birth defects and synergistics. The third issue is its effect on cognition both in the short and long terms. Gross also discusses the concept of "safe levels of drinking" or "threshold drinking" and how difficult it was to determine that level given the numerous variables such as gender, age, and other differences. He says that few people can drink as much in their later years as they did when they were young due to changes in the body's ability to handle alcohol. As we age the storage time of the alcohol is greater; its elimination is slower. The consensus of opinion, he concludes, is that two drinks a day is safe; more is too much. He also includes a broad range of advice such as measuring drinks, drinking wine and beer rather than hard liquor, drinking at meals, and drinking slowly.

088   Gurnack, Anne M., & Hoffman, Norman G. (1992). Elderly alcohol misuse. *International Journal of the Addictions, 27*(7), 869-878.

This study examined national data pertaining to problem drinking among the elderly. Subjects were 869 patients ages 60 and over admitted to treatment centers in 15 states during 1983-1985. Two-thirds of the sample were males and most were white. The data showed that some symptoms, such as those related to emotional distress, and employment status were associated with problem drinking for older adults. The findings also suggest that alcohol use throughout life may simply be carried into old age. The researchers noted a distinct pattern of drinking for older females in contrast to that of older males. They recommend that differences between the sexes and between early- and late-onset drinkers be considered when developing treatment and prevention programs.

089   Gurnack, Anne M., & Thomas, Jeanne L. (July, 1989). Behavioral factors related to elderly alcohol abuse: Research and policy issues. *International Journal of the Addictions, 24*(7), 641-654.

This paper reviews the existing literature with regard to elderly alcohol abuse and outlines future directions for research activity. The authors analyzed studies between 1965 and 1987 throughout the United States and England which had examined drinking patterns among the elderly. These studies investigated widely diverse samples from 24 to 2,746 people with alcoholic prevalence rates of 2.2% to 63%. The authors suggest future research is needed in alcohol use over the life course and how alcohol use patterns change over time. They call for a clearer differentiation between the early-onset and late-onset elderly problem drinkers.

090   Hartford, James T., & Samorajski, T. (Eds.). (1984). *Alcoholism in the elderly: Social and biomedical issues.* New York: Raven Press.
     This book includes articles by several medical and social sciences related to alcoholism and the elderly. Broad topics include sociology, biology and biochemistry, diagnosis and treatment, and emerging issues.

091   Hartford, James T., & Thienhaus, Ole J. (1984). Psychiatric aspects of alcoholism in geriatric patients. In James T. Hartford, & T. Samorajski (Eds.), *Alcoholism in the elderly: Social and biomedical issues* (pp. 253-262). New York: Raven Press.
     Alcohol abuse and dependence in the elderly tend to be seriously underestimated as a factor in presenting psycho-pathology and as a cause of many routine problems seen in emergency rooms and acute care clinics. The tendency to neglect alcoholism as part of the diagnosis is compounded by a lack of knowledge about the effects of alcohol on elderly patients. Problems seen in younger patients not seen in elderly e.g. absence from work, difficulties in the family, problems driving while intoxicated. The actual incidence of alcoholism in the elderly ranges from 15% to 25%. It is extremely difficult to differentiate between problems of aging and other medication conditions from alcoholism. Elderly patients who drink at all are more prone to alcohol-related problems than young people, including falls, memory loss, confusion, and sleep problems.

092   Haugland, Stanley. (June, 1989). Alcoholism and other drug dependencies. *Primary Care, 16*(2), 411-429.
     This article discusses major differences between the elderly and younger chemically dependent people. Haugland points out the increased number of addicted elderly due to the growth of the over 65 population. Differences of elderly drinkers include smaller amount consumed and increased sensitivity to the effects of alcohol; the greater number of elderly in the healthcare system; the greater number of prescriptions used; the tendency to pass off

symptoms of alcoholism as aging; and the tendency to downplay the seriousness of alcoholism and to recommend treatment for older people. The author presents a full discussion of prevalence, terms and definitions, historical considerations, prescription drug dependency, theoretical considerations, clinical presentations, addiction versus dependency, detoxification, and interventions.

093   Iliffe, Steve, Haines, Andrew, Booroff, Angela, Goldenberg, Eva, Morgan, Paula, & Gallivan, Stephen. (March, 1991). Alcohol consumption by elderly people: A general practice survey. *Age and Ageing, 20*(2), 120-123.

This study reports on the prevalence of alcohol consumption as measured by a modified version of the Health Survey Questionnaire and describes the relationships between frequency and quantity of alcohol consumption and cognitive impairment, depression, falls, contact with hospital specialists in outpatient clinics, and admission to hospital. The authors interviewed a random sample of 241 patients from General Practice registers in London. Fifty-one percent of men and 22% of women reported use of alcohol in the previous three months. Relationships between reported drinking status and age, score on a depression scale, falls in the previous three months, attendance at outpatient clinics or inpatient care in the previous year were not significant. In the men abstainers were significantly more likely to show cognitive impairment than were drinkers. Amongst those respondents who admitted to drinking within the previous three months, alcohol consumption was not associated with age, cognitive impairment and scores on the depression scale, and there was no association with falls, or with outpatient or inpatient care. Only three men (3.6%) and five women (3.2%) admitted consuming more than 21 and 14 units of alcohol per week, respectively. Only a minority of elderly people in this population drank alcohol with men more likely to drink than women. Only 3% drank above the "safe" limits. The data suggested that drinking alcohol was a characteristic of cognitively intact elderly people more so than those who are cognitively impaired.

094   James, O. F. W. (1984). The medical consequences of alcoholism in the elderly. In Neville Krasner, J. S. Madden, & Robin J. Walker (Eds.), *Alcohol related problems: Room for manoeuvre,* (pp. 147-157). New York: John Wiley & Sons.

James describes the range of physical disorders and diseases seen in people ages 65 and over caused by excess alcohol consumption which may lead to increased likelihood of death. Disorders and diseases either caused by or exacerbated by alcohol are liver disease, digestive disease, cardiovascular disease, organic brain syndromes, orthopedic/neurosurgical, drug interactions, and hypothermia. He also cites the increased likelihood of death from injuries such as suicide and accidents. He points out that while heavy alcohol consumption in the elderly is problematic, moderate consumption may be beneficial to many older people as a nighttime sedative, appetite stimulant, mood elevation, and improved mental functioning. James concludes that little is known about the epidemiology of the physical effects of alcohol.

095   Jensen, Gordon D., & Bellecci, Pauline. (1987). Alcohol and the elderly: Relationships to illness and smoking. *Alcohol and Alcoholism, 22*(2), 193-198.

This study focuses on the relationships varying amounts of alcohol use and physical, mental health, and life style variables. The subjects were 33 semi-independent living nonagenarian men and 32 men ages 65 to 75 of similar demographic characteristics, living at the California Veterans' Home. The younger group had a higher prevalence of alcohol abuse and higher current alcohol intake (p < .004). Higher alcohol intake (p < .004). In the younger group, higher alcohol intake was related to greater smoking of cigarettes. Alcohol tended to be related to an increased number of medical illnesses, and to increased use of major medications (p < .005). There was an interactive effect between classes of alcohol use and scores on a mental status examination used to assess cognitive function (p < .05). A past history of alcoholism and current pattern of moderate or heavy drinking was significantly associated with less healthy characteristics, more major medical illness, greater use of more medications and heavier cigarette smoking.

096   Klatsky, Abraham, L., Friedman, Gary D., Sieglaub, Abraham B., & Gerand, Marie J. (1977). Alcohol consumption among white, black, and Oriental men and women. *American Journal of Epidemiology, 105*, 311-323.

This paper reports health measurements of nondrinkers and drinkers of various alcoholic beverages by sex, race, and age. Data are also reported showing the association with alcohol consumption with other habits, educational attainment, and other variables. Subjects were 91,659 white, black, or Oriental men and women who recorded their alcohol consumption habits on health checkup questionnaires. Results of the data analysis showed that generally, men drank more than women, drinking was most prevalent among whites and least prevalent among Orientals, and the highest proportion of drinkers was found in the ages 20 to 29 and 30 to 39. Consumption of three plus drinks per day was most prevalent in ages 40 to 49 and 50 to 59. The proportion of nondrinkers diminished with increasing educational attainment. Alcohol use showed a strong positive association with cigarette smoking and a weaker positive association with coffee use. The authors concluded that age, sex, race, educational attainment, and smoking are potentially significant confounders of studies of alcohol use and health.

097   Kofoed, Lial L, Tolson, Robert L., Atkinson, Roland M., Turner, John A., & Toth, Rodger, F. (1984). Elderly groups in an alcoholism clinic. In Roland M. Atkinson, (Ed.), Alcohol and drug abuse in old age (pp. 35-48). Washington, DC: American Psychiatric Press, Inc.

This article describes a peer group treatment program for older alcoholic veterans. The program was open to any veteran accepted for outpatient alcoholism treatment who was on active military duty in 1945 or earlier. Groups met weekly for 90 minutes. The authors report data obtained from 42 participants ages 53 to 76 (mean age 61 years). The majority (n=39) were men. Onset of problem drinking varied from teens to 60s. Early-onset was associated with more family history of alcoholism. A majority of the referrals came from court diversion of arrested drinking drivers. Long term outcomes are not available; however, the authors' experience suggests that outpatient alcoholism treatment for the elderly might be successfully conducted in a variety of settings such as senior service centers, churches, or other social organizations as well as in alcoholic treatment programs.

098   Liberto, Joseph G., Oslin, David W., & Ruskin, Paul E. (October, 1992). Alcoholism in older persons: A review of the literature. *Hospital and Community Psychiatry, 43*(10), 975-984.

In this paper, the authors review the literature on the epidemiology, physical consequences, and treatment of alcohol use and abuse among elderly people. They present a summary of the findings from 21 studies conducted between 1960 and 1990. Most samples were ages 60 and over. Sample sizes varied from 30 to 1,509. Abstainers ranged from 31% to 58%. The percentage of daily drinkers reported in four studies ranged from 10% to 22%. The authors report that the most consistent findings of cross-sectional and longitudinal studies are that the quantity and frequency of alcohol consumption is higher in elderly men than in elderly women, as is the prevalence of alcohol-related problems. Most studies show a decrease with age in consumption and alcohol-related problems among heavy drinkers. Longitudinal studies show no changes in consumption among light drinkers. Elderly persons with lower incomes consume less alcohol than those with higher incomes. Hospitalized and outpatient populations have more problem drinkers, and the elderly alcoholic is at greater risk for medical and psychiatric comorbidity. About one-third to one-half of elderly alcoholics experience the onset of problem drinking in middle or late life. Outcomes seem to be better for those who have late-onset drinking and may be improved for those treated in same-age rather than mixed-age groups.

099   Lichtenberg, Peter A., Gibbons, T. Ann, Nanna, Michael J., & Blumenthal, Frank. (1993). The effects of age and gender on the prevalence and detection of alcohol abuse in elderly medical inpatients. *Clinical Gerontologist, 13*(3), 17-28.

This study investigated age and gender effects on alcohol abuse in the older medical patient. Subjects were 168 consecutive admission of patients ages 60 and over seen by the primary author on either the stroke or geriatric unit between January and October 1991. As part of the evaluation, he administered the CAGE. Physician detection was assessed by a blind chart review at least one week subsequent to admission. Overall, 17% of patients were alcohol abusers. Data analysis revealed significant age and gender effects. The young–old patients (ages 60 to 74) had a much higher prevalence of abuse than did old–old patients (ages 75 and over). Men had a higher prevalence of abuse than did women. Physician detection was highly related to the patient's gender. Over half of the male abusers were correctly detected but no alcohol abusing woman was detected.

100   Maddox, George, Robbins, Lee N., & Rosenberg, Nathan (Eds.). (1986). *Nature and extent of alcohol problems among the elderly.* New York: Springer.

This volume is one of a series of research monographs from NIAAA which includes current information on topics relevant to alcohol abuse and alcoholism. It includes the text of a workshop on alcohol-related problems among the elderly. Individual chapters present position papers, results of studies, panel discussions, and reaction papers.

101   Magruder-Habib, Kathryn, Harris, Katherine E., & Fraker, Glynn G. (1982). Validation of the Veterans Alcoholism Screening Test. *Journal of Studies on Alcohol, 43*(9), 910-926.

This study compared the Veterans Alcoholism Screening Test (VAST) and the Michigan Alcoholism Screening Test (MAST). The authors administered the VAST and the MAST to a sample of 118 pairs of ambulatory care patients and their relatives. The VAST was found to be a more valid, useful, and accurate indicator of alcoholism than the MAST when distinguishing between current and former alcoholics.

102   Magruder-Habib, Kathryn, Saltz, Constance C., & Barron, Patricia M. (December, 1986). Age-related patterns of alcoholism among veterans in ambulatory care. *Hospital and Community Psychiatry, 37*(12), 1251-1255.

The purpose of this study was to determine the relationship between patients' scores on the Veterans Alcoholism Screening Test (VAST) and an independent assessment of patient status. A trained administrator administered the VAST to 118 outpatients ages 22 to 87 (mean age 59 years). The Michigan Alcoholism Screening Test (MAST) was also administered. These data showed the VAST was a more valid indicator of alcoholism than the MAST based on agreement between patient and relative responses. The VAST also provided more information as to drinking problems in different periods of life. The prevalence of alcoholism ever in a person's life was 50% using the patient data and 42.7% using relative data. A copy of the VAST is included as an appendix.

103   Malcolm, M. T. (1984). Problem drinking in the elderly. In Neville Krasner, J. S. Madden, & Robin J. Walker (Eds.), *Alcohol related problems: Room for manoeuvre* (pp. 139-146). New York: John Wiley & Sons.

Over a 2.5-year period, Malcolm conducted a study to examine the drinking patterns and medications used among 191 patients ages 65 to 95. Subjects were interviewed in their own homes in England. They took an average of three medications; 10% took no medications. Of the 191 subjects, 69 (36%) reported some use of alcohol. Three groups of drinkers emerged: the occasional drinker where there was no alcohol problem (n=41); the frequent drinker where alcohol influenced the patient's health (n=9); and the abusive drinker (n=19). Abusive drinking involved regular drunkenness, falling, arrests, and drunken injuries. Malcolm concluded that problem drinking among the elderly was an under-recognized problem that needed more attention.

104   Mangion, D. M., Platt, J. S., & Syam, V. (September, 1992). Alcohol and acute medical admission of elderly people. *Age and Ageing, 21*(5), 363-368.

This prospective study examined the prevalence and determinants of alcohol abuse and alcohol-related medical admissions among a sample of elderly patients using an alcohol-intake history, caregiver interviews, CAGE questionnaire, and laboratory tests. The subjects were 539 elderly patients (mean age 77.3 years; 275 men and 264 women). Results indicated 42 patients (7.8%, 36 men and 6 women) were classified as alcohol abusers; 41 were identified by an alcohol intake history and one by a positive response to the CAGE questionnaire; none was identified by laboratory screening alone. Abuse was higher among men than women; 50.6% of the men and 83.7% of the women were abstainers or occasional drinkers. Men who reported drinking more in the past had reduced their drinking because of ill health (36%), loss of social contact (28%), financial difficulties (19%), a feeling that alcohol was impairing health (4%), or no specific reason (13%). Of the admissions, 13 were due directly to alcohol intoxication/falls, delirium tremens, self-neglect, neuropathy, and self-poisoning by alcohol and drugs. Compared with an alcohol intake history, the CAGE and laboratory screening showed good specificity but poor sensitivity; only the CAGE questionnaire showed good positive predictive value. The authors concluded that while the sensitivities of the CAGE questionnaire and laboratory screening were too low to be clinically useful, an alcohol intake history may allow for a significant opportunity in preventive medicine with the elderly.

105   Merrill, Mundle, Kraft, Philip Graham, Gordon, Margaret, Holmes, Mary Marrs, & Walker, Bobbie. (1990). *Chemically dependent older adults: How do we treat them?* Center City, MN: Hazelden.

Chemically dependent older adults can be successfully treated. The authors describe the process of conducting an assessment and an intervention with a chemically dependent older adult. They discuss the issues that need to be understood and considered in choosing a treatment method suited to individual older adults. This text also deals with continuing care and family issues relative to helping chemically addicted older adults.

106   Meyers, Allan R., Golman, Eli, Hingson, Ralph, & Scotch, Norman. (1981-82). Evidence for cohort or generational differences in the drinking behavior of older adults. *International Journal of Aging and Human Development, 14,* 31-43.

This cross-sectional study investigated drinking patterns among older adults. The authors surveyed 928 older Bostonians. Data analysis revealed a negative correlation between age and alcohol consumption. The "old–old," people ages 75 and over, were more likely to abstain and less likely to drink in any quantity than the "younger–old," ages 65 to 74. Levels of abstinence were highest among females, Jews, blacks, and people with no formal education beyond high school. Approximately 53% of the group were abstainers; 26% drank less than one drink per day. The most popular beverage was liquor (43%) with wine second (27%). Only 9% said they usually drank beer.

107   Midanik, Lorraine T., & Room, Robin. (1992). The epidemiology of alcohol consumption. *Alcohol Health & Research World, 16*(3), 183-190.

This article discusses the public health perspective on drinking patterns in the population at large. The authors explain how data regarding alcohol consumption are collected and how results need to be interpreted. They also discuss method of conducting surveys of drinking practices and explain advantages and disadvantages of this method as compared to consumption statistics. They discuss problems in data collection due to variability in volume, frequency, and patterns of drinking. Included are data on drinking patterns by gender, age, education level, and family income of the United States general adult population obtained in 1990. The survey found that 71% of the population drink alcohol at least occasionally and 10% drink daily. Among Americans ages 60 and over, the proportion using alcohol was found to be 66% with 16% drinking daily.

108   Miller, Norman S., Belkin, Beth M., & Gold, Mark S. (March-April, 1991). Alcohol and drug dependence among the elderly: Epidemiology, diagnosis, and treatment. *Comprehensive Psychiatry, 32*(2), 153-65.

This paper reports the findings of the Epidemiologic Catchment Area Program which assessed the prevalence of alcohol and drug dependence using DSM-III-R criteria by assessing subjects in five major United States cities. The authors report that prevalence rates were higher for younger than for older ages and for men than women. For men, lifetime prevalence was 14% for people ages 65 and over and 1.5% for women. The authors discuss the results of the study in depth and report features of geriatric addiction and common patterns of use of alcohol and drugs, psychiatric complications, etiology and pathogenesis, differential diagnosis, the relationship of alcohol and drug dependence and dementia, and treatment. They conclude that the prognosis for untreated alcoholism and drug dependence in the elderly is poor. Treatment is required for permanent remission.

109   Minnis, John R. (Spring, 1988). Toward an understanding of alcohol abuse among the elderly: A sociological perspective. *Journal of Alcohol and Drug Education, 33*(3), 32-40.

This paper reviews some of the demographics of aging and alcohol abuse among the aged. The author suggests that the social control perspective of deviance may be useful in investigating alcohol abuse among the elderly. This theory assumes that deviant acts result when an individual's bond to society is weak or broken. Using this theory, Minnis hypothesizes that the greater the attachment to conventional others, the greater the commitment to conventional goals or aspirations, the greater the involvement in conventional activities, and the greater the beliefs in the moral validity of conventional norms, the less likely is the elderly person to engage in alcohol abuse. These points need to be investigated in future research.

110   Mishara, Brian L., & Kastenbaum, Robert. (1980). *Alcohol and old age.* New York: Grune & Stratton.

The authors of this book, through explanation of various studies and statistical information, draw conclusions about the elderly and their use of alcohol. First, because alcohol use appears to be more moderate in the elderly population, and because that moderate use has been linked to only a few detrimental effects, the authors suggest there is no evidence to support viewing alcohol as an unqualified menace to the elderly. Second, although moderate use could be of positive value in some elderly, heavy drinking continues to pose a serious risk to health and well-being. The authors also include a list of recommendations for outreach and treatment of elderly alcoholics based on their findings.

111   Mishara, Brian L, & Kastenbaum, Robert. (1980). Problem drinking. In Brian L. Mishara, & Robert Kastenbaum (Eds.), *Alcohol and old age* (pp. 61-84). New York: Grune & Stratton.

The authors discuss the nature of "problem drinking" in old age. Most clients with drinking problems, in their experience, neither realize they have a problem nor admit to it. They list symptoms of drinking problems as: symptoms developed as a result of drinking such as hangovers, blackouts, memory loss and shakes; psychological dependence on alcohol; health problems related to alcohol use; financial problems related to alcohol use; interpersonal problems with a spouse, relatives, friends, or neighbors related to alcohol use; problems on the job as a result of drinking; belligerence associated with drinking; and problems with the police or the law as a result of drinking. They note that people may have any of the symptoms or problems without anyone knowing they are related to alcohol use. From their review of studies of older alcoholics and epidemiological studies of drinking among the elderly, the authors conclude that the problem may be more wide-spread that previous studies have shown due to current definitions of problem drinking which may not fit the elderly, the difficulty in identifying characteristics of elderly people who may be drinking secretly, and the limitations of samples providing data for most existing studies.

112   Mishara, Brian L., & McKim, William. (March, 1993). Methodological issues in surveying older persons concerning drug use. *International Journal of Addictions, 28*(4), 305-326.

This article reviews methodological issues in surveying the use of medications, over-the-counter drugs, alcohol, caffeine, tobacco, and recreational drugs among older persons. The authors conclude that empirical verifications do not support the belief that surveys involving older persons are less valid than those with other groups (due to memory loss, etc.). They recommend considering other factors related to reduced validity such as educational levels, cohort characteristics, and time of measurement. They believe that people with dementia and institutional residents are often needlessly excluded. They suggest several methods for improving validity in studies with older subjects including sampling techniques, proxy respondents, administration and instrumentation, and interviewer variables. They recommend cross-validating data from surveys by using several concurrent methods. They point out that instruments developed with younger subjects may be inappropriate or invalid with elders.

113   Molgaard, Craig A., Nakamura, Chester M., Stanford, E. Percil, Peddecord, K. Michael, & Morton, Deborah J. (August, 1990). Prevalence of alcohol consumption among older persons. *Journal of Community Health, 15*(4), 239-251.

This cross-sectional study investigated the prevalence of alcohol use among a randomly chosen population ages 45 and over. The study sample (N=2,105) showed statistically significant drinking differences between whites (n=819), blacks (n=629), and Mexican-Americans (n=657). Overall, the highest prevalence of drinking occurred among the white elderly. The common belief that socioeconomic conditions are inversely associated with a high prevalence of drinking was not supported in this sample. Statistically significant differences in age-specific and sex-specific percent prevalences of alcohol intake were also found. There was a generally decreasing prevalence of alcohol consumption with advancing age, which existed regardless of ethnicity.

114   Moos, Rudolf H., Mertens, Jennifer R., & Brennan, Penny L. (July, 1993). Patterns of diagnosis and treatment among late-middle-aged and older substance abuse patients. *Journal of Studies on Alcohol, 54*(4), 479-488.

This study compares the rate of diagnosis and treatment of elderly problem drinkers with the same rate among younger patients. Subjects included more than 22,000 Veterans Administration hospital patients admitted during 1987. More than 23% of those admitted for substance abuse problems were ages 55 or over, and most of this older group had multiple health problems. Over 90% of this group had alcohol-related problems. Data analysis revealed that the older substance abuse patients were less likely to receive treatment geared toward their specific substance abuse or psychiatric problems than the younger patients. Older group members were more likely to receive treatment geared toward medical problems. The authors suggest a need for more specific programs of treatment geared toward the substance abuse problems of older adults, rather than relying on treatment solely related to their various medical problems.

115   Mulford, Harold A., & Fitzgerald, J. L. (November, 1982). Elderly versus younger problem drinker profiles: Do they indicate a

need for special programs for the elderly? *Journal of Studies on Alcohol, 53*(11), 601-610.

The purpose of this study was to compare younger persons (ages 18 to 54) with two overlapping elderly age groups (ages 55 and over and 65 and over) to determine whether special programs were needed for the elderly. The sample consisted of 1,430 people whose driving license had been revoked and who were contacted by phone or mail. Although there were several statistically significant differences between the elderly and younger problem drinkers, there was as much, or more, heterogeneity within the elderly groups as there were differences between the elderly and their younger counterparts. Also, the descriptive profile of these at-large elderly problem drinkers differed, depending on whether their alcohol abuse was early- or late-onset. The authors concluded that age-specific treatment for the elderly was not justified.

116   Office for Substance Abuse Prevention National Training System. (1991). *The physician does make a difference: Recognizing the faces of alcohol and drug abuse* [videotape]. Rockville, MD: National Clearinghouse for Alcohol and Drug Information.

This videotape illustrates the problems associated with physician diagnoses of alcohol or drug abuse. There are an estimated 18 million problem drinkers in the United States. An estimated 20% of all patients have a problem with alcohol or other drugs. The video uses examples from a training program at Brown University that teaches medical students to include alcohol or drug questions in a routine history-taking with a minimum of discomfort and conflict. A supplementary pamphlet gives suggestions for viewing the tape and describes the major points emphasized in the presentation.

117   Olsen-Noll, Cynthia G., & Bosworth, Michael F. (April, 1989). Alcohol abuse in the elderly. *American Family Physician, 39*(4), 173-179.

This article discusses classification and characteristics of elderly alcoholics, and physiologic consequences and why they go unnoticed. The authors conclude that alcoholism is often difficult to recognize in the elderly, that information about alcoholic behavior cannot always be accurately extrapolated to older drinkers, and that consequences of alcohol abuse and responses to treatment may be quite different in young and elderly alcoholics. They recommend that physicians focus treatment on such day-to-day problems as loneliness, loss of independence and declining health and use gentle persistence to guide patients to an awareness of their problem.

118 **Osgood, Nancy J. (1988). Identifying and treating the geriatric alcoholic.** *Geriatric Medicine Today,* **7(8), 53-57.**
This article provides a brief overview of the problem of geriatric alcoholism, discusses major factors in elderly alcoholism, identifies clues and warnings, and offers hints and suggestions on treating the geriatric alcoholic. Osgood states that alcoholism in the elderly is an under recognized, under diagnosed, and under reported illness. She points out the difficulty in diagnosing this problem in an elderly individual because many of the psychological, physical, and behavioral symptoms of the disease mimic those of other degenerative disorders. She observes that the physician is in the best position to identify the geriatric alcoholic, who often successfully hides excessive drinking from family and friends and should, therefore, be aware of the various mental, physical, and social warning signs of alcoholism, such as depression, and the high–risk groups susceptible to alcoholism. She offers suggestions for treating the elderly alcoholic include treating the concomitant depression as the primary problem.

119 **Osgood, Nancy J., Wood, Helen E., & Parham, Iris A. (1995).** *Alcoholism and aging: An annotated bibliography and review.* **Westport, CT: Greenwood Press.**
This annotated bibliography and review lists over 300 works on the subject of alcohol and aging. The authors include bibliographies, overview articles, books and book chapters, empirical studies, and miscellaneous works.

120 **Scherr, Paul A., LaCroix, Andrea Z., Wallace, Robert B., Berkman, Lisa, Curb, J. David, Cornoni-Huntley, Joan, Evans, Denis A., & Hennekens, Charles H. (July, 1992). Light to moderate alcohol consumption and mortality in the elderly.** *Journal of the American Geriatrics Society,* **40(7), 651-657.**
This prospective study investigated the relationship of low to moderate alcohol consumption with cardiovascular mortality in the elderly. Subjects were population-based cohorts of men and women (ages 65 and over) in three populations. Subjects with prior myocardial infarction, stroke, or cancer, as well as those lacking alcohol consumption data, were excluded from statistical analyses leaving 2,694 subjects in East Boston, Massachusetts, 2,293 subjects in Iowa, and 1,904 subjects in New Haven, Connecticut. The

authors conclude that the relationship of low to moderate alcohol consumption with reduced total and cardiovascular mortality, documented in middle age in other studies, also occur in older populations.

121   **Schonfeld, Lawrence, & Dupree, Larry W. (November, 1991). Antecedents of drinking for early- and late-onset elderly alcohol abusers.** *Journal of Studies on Alcohol,* 52(6), 587-592.

This study compared antecedents to recent drinking for two groups of elderly alcohol abusers in a treatment program. Early-onset alcohol abusers (n=23) were matched with late-onset alcohol abusers (n=23) according to age and sex. The most frequently reported antecedents to preadmission drinking behavior for both groups were depression, loneliness and lack of social support. Early-onset subjects were more likely to have changed residence, were intoxicated more often, and experienced more severe levels of depression and anxiety. Late-onset subjects had greater life satisfaction and motivation for treatment. The authors suggest treatment implications.

122   **Scott, Robert B. (June, 1989). Alcohol effects in the elderly.** *Comprehensive Therapy,* 15(6), 8-12.

This article describes the cultural patterns of alcohol use and reviews alcohol's metabolic and pathologic effects on older people. Scott states that alcohol is a potent drug that should be included in the medication history of the patient. He suggests that since typical clues may not be present physicians need to be alert to the possibility of alcohol abuse by the elderly. He points out that alcohol has a greater dose-related effect in elderly persons because of their decreased total body water, which leads to persistently higher blood alcohol levels, and that alcohol causes unique kinds of brain damage, a fact that may aggravate the clinical symptoms of dementia such as Alzheimer's disease. Because alcohol potentiates the sedating effects of many drugs acting on the central nervous system, elderly patients should be cautioned concerning the use of alcohol and drugs.

123   **Smart, Reginald G., & Adlaf, Edward M. (July-August, 1988). Alcohol and drug use among the elderly: Trends in use and characteristics of users.** *Canadian Journal of Public Health,* 79(4), 236-242.

This study examined trends in alcohol and drug use among the elderly and demographic and structural factors associated with use. Data were derived from four cross-sectional surveys conducted between 1976 and 1984. Overall the results indicated no dramatic trends in use. Males were most likely to report frequent alcohol use, females were more likely to report sleeping pill use and prevalence of tranquilizer use. Data were collected from 1976 to 1977 and again in 1982 to 1984. Proportion of abstainers reported were 43.3% and 35.4%. Proportions reporting sleeping pill use were 18.4% and 14.0%. Tranquilizer use was reported by 13.1% and 13.6% of the subjects.

124 Smart, Reginald G., & Liban, Carolyn B. (April-June, 1981). **Predictors of problem drinking among elderly, middle-aged and youthful drinkers.** *Journal of Psychoactive Drugs, 13*(2), 153-163.

This paper presents data and analyses related to age as a predictor of drinking problems. Subjects were 1,013 adults ages 18 and over who were interviewed in 1978 in Canada. There were 142 subjects ages 60 and over. Age was negatively associated with alcohol dependency symptoms. Three variables predicted alcohol dependency in the older group of subjects: sex, frequency of drinking, and volume of consumption. The elderly problem drinker was more difficult to predict than younger drinkers. The elderly problem drinker was most likely to be male, born outside of Canada, not retired, in the lower income and socioeconomic groups and drinking several times a week though not in particularly large quantities. The authors conclude that the elderly problem drinkers are difficult to predict because of lower consumption rates which are less likely to lead to many of the symptoms included in the dependency measure.

125 Smith, Gordon S., & Kraus, Jess F. (1988). **Alcohol and residential, recreational, and occupational injuries: A review of the epidemiologic evidence.** *Annual Review of Public Health, 9,* 99-121.

This paper reviews the role of alcohol in residential, recreational, and occupational settings and suggests why these situations present different environments in which to control alcohol-related injuries. The authors summarize literature on the subject of alcohol and nonvehicular injuries in the general population published since 1960. Findings are presented related to alcohol and injury risk, residential injuries (falls, burns and fires, poisoning, suffocation, firearm, drowning, falling objects, electrocution, hypothermia), recreational injuries (drowning, snowmobiling, skiing, spectator sports, organized sports),

Aviation and related recreational activities, and occupational injuries. The authors conclude that despite the numerous methodological problems with present studies that there is considerable evidence that alcohol is involved with a wide variety of activities and related injuries. They point out specific injury types where the elderly are at highest risk such as falls and burns and fires.

126   Stall, Ron. (May, 1987). Research issues concerning alcohol consumption among aging populations. *Drug and Alcohol Dependence, 19*(3), 195-213.

This comprehensive review of the literature focuses on patterns of alcohol use and how they change across the life course rather than on the extent of problem drinking among the elderly. The research concerning alcohol use and aging is reviewed to highlight reasons for change and stability in alcohol consumption for people past age 40 which Stall identifies as the second half of life. He defines elderly as those ages 65 and over.

127   Sulsky, Sandra I., Jacques, Paul F., Otradovec, Constant L., Hartz, Stuart C., & Russell, Robert M. (August, 1990). Descriptors of alcohol consumption among noninstitutionalized nonalcoholic elderly. *Journal of the American College of Nutrition, 9*(4), 326-331.

This paper describes relationships between reported alcohol consumption and selected sociodemographic and health variables. Subjects were 204 men and 367 women ages 60 to 95 examined as part of a nutritional status survey of elderly. In this sample, 53% of men and 44% of women reported drinking at least two grams of alcohol per week. Men were more likely to drink than women, and the level of alcohol consumption decreased with age. Drinking was positively associated with education ($p < .01$) and negatively associated with recent medical care ($p < .01$), history of mental illness ($p < .05$), and denture use ($p < .05$). Among drinkers, reported alcohol intake was higher for subjects under age 70 ($p < .01$), males ($p < .01$), the college educated ($p < .01$), and smokers ($p < .05$). Level of alcohol intake was lower for those who had received medical care in the year preceding study participation ($p < .05$). Identical results were observed for alcohol intake expressed as percent of total calories. Intake ranged from 3.8% of total calories among subjects ages 80 and over to 6.2% of total calories among ages 60 to 69.

128 Tucker, Jalie A., Gavornik, Michele G., Vuchinich, Rudy E., Rudd, Edmund J., & Harris, Carole V. (1989). Predicting the drinking behavior of older adults from questionnaire measure of alcohol consumption. *Addictive Behaviors, 14*(6), 655-658.

This study investigated the relationship between three questionnaire measures of alcohol consumption and self-monitoring reports of drinking in the natural environment. Subjects were 83 normal drinkers ages 60 and over. Following questionnaire administration subjects recorded their alcohol consumption each day for up to three months. Collaterals verified subjects' self-monitoring reports. Questionnaire scores and self-monitoring reports of frequency and quantity of alcohol consumption were generally well correlated. Regression analyses showed the Questionnaire Measure of Habitual Alcohol Use to be the best predictor of both drinking frequency and quantity. The authors discuss measurement issues related to the use of verbal reports of alcohol consumption with elderly drinkers.

129 Widner, Sabina, & Zeichner, Amos. (1991). Alcohol abuse in the elderly: Review of epidemiology research and treatment. *Clinical Gerontologist, 11*(1), 3-18.

This literature review critically evaluates current research on alcohol abuse, illicit drug abuse, and the treatment of alcohol abuse in the elderly. Research is presented related to prevalence of alcohol use among the elderly, identifying the elderly problem drinker, types of elderly problem drinkers, the phenomena referred to as "maturing out of problem drinking," alcohol and physiological processes in the elderly, and alcohol treatment in the elderly. The authors conclude that elderly problem drinkers constitute approximately 10% of the population. They are divided into two groups: early onset (two thirds) and late onset (one third). The elderly drinking problem can be expected to increase in the future due to the increased number of people ages 65 and over and the increased number of people in younger cohorts who use alcohol. They call for increasing the data base relative to demographic variables in the elderly alcoholic population and additional focus on the underlying causes of alcohol abuse. Well-controlled longitudinal studies are needed to establish a comprehensive model of the interactive effects of genetic predisposition, personality-based attributes, and life stresses on the development of geriatric substance abuse. Studies are also needed to resolve many issues related to treatment services.

130   Willenbring, Mark L, Christensen, Kathy J., Spring, William D, Jr., & Rasmussen, Reva. (1987). Alcoholism screening in the elderly. *Journal of the American Geriatrics Society, 35,* 864–869.

The purpose of this study was to validate the Michigan Alcoholism Screen Test (MAST), the Brief MAST (BMAST), the Short MAST (SMAST), and the UMAST (unit scoring) with a population of elderly. Subjects were 52 hospitalized elderly male alcoholics and 33 nonalcoholic controls. The authors found that the MAST and UMAST showed excellent sensitivity and specificity, while the SMAST was less specific, and the BMAST less sensitive and less specific. Factor structure of the two brief versions was similar to that found in younger alcoholics, suggesting that symptom constellation is not necessarily different in the elderly. They recommend the use of the MAST or UMAST for screening for alcoholism in the elderly.

131   Williams, Millree. (Spring 1984). Alcohol and the elderly: An overview. *Alcohol Health & Research World, 8*(3), 3–9, 52.

This article discusses a number of topics related to the elderly and heavy or problem drinking and reports NIAAA data estimating that approximately 10% of elderly men and 2% of elderly females are problem drinkers. While Williams acknowledges that the elderly who drink heavily appear to decrease their consumption as they age, he points out that they also show a decreased tolerance to alcohol. He describes the difficulty in identifying problem use among the elderly because the usual indicators such as problems with the law or jobs are not as applicable. He also states that physicians misdiagnose alcoholism in the elderly because the symptoms are similar to other conditions associated with aging and adverse drug reactions. He cites evidence that a certain number of elderly people develop problems in late life. Williams also discusses treatment and prevention efforts.

132   Zimberg, Sheldon. (1979). Alcohol and the elderly. In David M. Petersen, Frank J. Whittington, & Barbara P. Payne (Eds.), *Drugs and the elderly* (pp. 28–40). Springfield, IL: Charles C. Thomas.

Zimberg's analysis of 15 empirical studies of alcohol use among the elderly conducted between 1965 and 1974 led him to conclude that alcohol abuse among that age group might be underdiagnosed and underreported. In addition to prevalence studies, he cites evidence from hospital records and police records that alcoholism is a significant geriatric problem. He cites evidence from one study that as many as a quarter of elderly alcoholics may become alcoholic after age 60. He reports that many physicians often prescribe alcohol for elderly patients who have experienced loss of appetite or insomnia and that these symptoms are often caused by depression. In his view there are better drugs for depression than alcohol. He also states that physicians in general have been unwilling to recognize the problems of alcoholism and make a diagnosis. He notes that physicians have a general feeling of hopelessness about treating alcoholics and that those feelings are even more pronounced in relation to elderly patients.

3

Burns and Scalds

Fire and burn injuries are the fifth leading cause of accidental death for people ages 55 and over. The majority of these deaths occur in house fires. Other causes of burn injuries are hot water scalds, contact burns from appliances, and mouth burns from hot foods. The articles in this chapter present information regarding prevalence of injuries in this category as well as prevalence of burns related to specific hazards. Many articles discuss fire safety issues. Articles and publications are also included that address prevention issues.

133   Baptiste, Mark, & Feck, Gerald. (1980). **Preventing tap water burns.** *American Journal of Public Health, 70*(7), 727-729.
      Based on a 1974-1975 survey of hospital records in upstate New York, the authors estimate that 347 tap water burns will require inpatient treatment annually, with children and the elderly at the highest risk. The number and severity of burns from tap water makes this type of accident an important prevention priority. Reducing the temperature of household hot water supplies could be a practical and effective prevention measure.

134   *Blueprint for fire safety: A special program planning guide on basic fire safety lessons for senior citizens.* (Spring, 1988). Washington, DC: Federal Emergency Management Agency.
      This book outlines fire safety programs for senior citizens. It describes ways for the elderly to prevent fires and burns related to cooking and smoking, and to treat minor burns and scalds. The

authors also give suggestions for planning pre- and posttests, group reviews, fire safety skits, and contests to reinforce the fire safety message.

135   Blye, Phillip, & Yess, James P. (November-December, 1987). Firesafety in elderly housing. *Fire Journal, 81*(6), 28-30; 75-76.

This article describes the National Fire Protection Association's (NFPA) Simplified Fire Safety System (SFSS), in which the NFPA has modified general fire protection principles to target specialized buildings such as correctional facilities, hotels, hospitals, and board and care homes. Overall fire protection goals for facilities that house elderly people are life safety and property protection. These goals may be achieved in several steps: by modifying or building facilities to eliminate uncontrolled sources of heat that may start a fire, by controlling fuel sources or installing fire and smoke barriers that can prevent the spread of fire, by implementing adequate evacuation plans, and by having the appropriate methods for detecting and suppressing fires. The authors explain each of these steps in detail, and give practical suggestions specifically applying to elderly housing facilities.

136   Brodzka, Wanda, Thornhill, Herbert L., & Howard, Sally. (November, 1985). Burns: Causes and risk factors. *Archives of Physical and Medical Rehabilitation, 66*(11), 746-752.

This retrospective study examined the characteristics of an adult burn population to correlate the circumstances of their injuries and the incidence of pre-burn risk factors. Researchers reviewed the records of 277 people (mean age 44.5 years) who had been hospitalized for a burn injury over a five-year period. Of these subjects, 78% were black, 62% were men, and 74% were burned at home. The most common cause of burns was flames (44.8%), followed by scalds (28.5%), and chemicals (9.7%). Alcohol abuse was the most common risk factor (28%), followed by being ages 60 and over (20%). Other factors that increased the likelihood of injury included drug abuse, physical or mental illness, and living alone. The authors suggest that proper housing and simple safety practices (such as not smoking in bed or setting water heaters at a safe temperature) could have prevented most of the injuries.

137   Burn prevention and treatment tips. (March, 1992). *American Family Physician, 45*(5), 1331-1332.

The American Academy of Family Physicians prepared this list of tips for family physicians to use and distribute to their patients. The recommendations include safe water heater temperatures, ways to treat minor burns, and tips for wound and dressing care. The tips may be reproduced free of charge for nonprofit, educational purposes.

138   Canter, David (Ed.). (1990). *Fires & human behavior: Second edition.* London: David Fulton Publishers.

This text presents several chapters on the subject of human behavior in fire. Of special interest are the chapters on the concept of panic, a survey on behavior in fires, a studies of fire in hospitals, and fires in nursing homes. A chapter written by the editor provides suggestions in training people to avoid disasters.

139   Conley, Christopher J., & Fahy, Rita F. (May-June, 1994). Who dies in fires in the United States? *NFPA Journal, 88*(3), 99-106.

The authors use statistics on fire deaths in the United States to identify those at highest risk and to find out what conditions decrease the risk. The very young and the elderly are at highest risk for fire deaths. The fire death rate for children ages 5 and under is more than twice the national average. For the elderly, the death rates increase with age: ages 65 and over, the rate is twice the national average; for those ages 75 and over, it is almost three times the national average; and for those ages 85 and over, it is four times the national average. Males, the physically and mentally handicapped, the homeless, those living in poverty, smokers, those using alcohol or other drugs, children playing with fire or setting fires, and residents of homes with security measures that hamper escape are also at high risk for fire deaths. Conditions that reduce the risk include public fire education programs, smoke detectors, and sprinklers.

140   Demling, Robert H. (November 28, 1985). Burns. *New England Journal of Medicine, 313*(22), 1389-1398.

The author reviews the prevalence and epidemiology of burn injuries in the United States, which has the highest incidence of burns among all industrialized countries. A United States citizen has a 1 in 70 chance of being hospitalized for a burn injury in his or her lifetime. Only motor vehicle accidents cause more accidental deaths. Most burns occur among children ages 1 to 5, of which a majority are caused by scalds from hot liquids. The elderly are the second highest risk group. The author suggests that although little has been done to prevent burn injuries, much has been done to improve the victim's chance of survival and recovery. The article presents detailed information on treatment, including the immediate response, continuing care for infection, wound management, and skin grafting.

141   **Electric-blanket fires. (June 6, 1963).** *New England Journal of Medicine, 268*(23), 1308.

Electric blanket fires have been the cause of 7,000 fires in the United Kingdom. Sixty-one persons were injured and two of these died. The electric blankets were either defective or improperly used. Two of the many models of electric blankets on the market have built-in safety systems that make them safe to use, but they are relatively expensive. Standards are being revised for the making of the blankets. Reliable figures on electric blanket and heating pad fires are hard to obtain in the United States, because minor incidents are not usually reported by the local fire departments. There were 18 reported fires during May, 1955-December, 1960; 2 were caused by heating pads, and 16 by electric blankets. Electric blankets and heating pads do not appear to cause the same amount of fires in the United States as they do in the United Kingdom, unless the system of reporting fires is more effective in United Kingdom than in the United States. However, these devices should be manufactured and used as carefully as other electrical equipment such as irons, heaters, or stoves.

142   *Fire in the United States (7th Ed.).* **(1990). Emmitsburg, MD: U. S. Fire Administration.**

This book is a report from the United States Fire Administration giving a statistical overview of the fire problem in the United States. The report is designed to direct fire prevention programs, to serve as a model for local fire data gathering, and to provide a foundation from which to evaluate fire safety programs. The data are analyzed to identify fire risk factors and high-risk groups, and to predict trends in fire injury, loss, and death.

143   **Gerard, Warren. (July 28, 1980). Nursing homes: Everybody's nightmare.** *MacLean's, 93*(30), 17-21.

This article describes a nursing home fire in Toronto, Ontario, Canada. An 85-year-old resident had been smoking in his room (which was prohibited at the facility), which resulted in a fire that killed 21 people. All but one of the fatalities were due to smoke inhalation. The author discusses the problems of residents in Canada's licensed and unlicensed care facilities, including overcrowding, improper use of medication, poor supervision, and inadequate standards and inspections for safety hazards.

144   Groner, Norman E. (May, 1986). *Fire safety in board and care homes.* Rockville, MD: Project Share.

This manual is based on the safety margin principle, which states that, when a fire occurs, there must be more time available to carry out the fire emergency plan than actually needed. In other words, determining how much time each emergency plan takes. will enable staff to choose a strategy based on how much time is available. The manual covers both escape and refuge strategies, explaining how this safety margin affects each approach. The book also describes ways to increase the safety margin (including decreasing the time needed and increasing the time available), planning tips, and ways to implement fire planning strategies.

145   Hall, John R., Jr. (January-February, 1989). The latest statistics on U. S. home smoke detectors. *Fire Journal, 83*(1), 39-41.

This article discusses the importance of home smoke detectors in saving lives. Homes that are poor or headed by the elderly or less educated are less likely to use smoke detectors. The use of smoke detectors can cut the risk of death from fire in half. The most common factor influencing nonoperational smoke detectors is having dead or missing batteries. The author recommends that the public be educated to properly install, use, and test smoke detectors in their own homes.

146   Hall, John R., Jr. (July-August, 1990). The elderly, the sick, and health care facilities. *Fire Journal, 84*(4), 32-42.

The author describes elderly adults (ages 65 and over) as one of the most distinguishable groups at high risk of fire deaths because there are more elderly people than preschool children (the only other group with a comparable fire death risk), because they are the fastest-growing population in the United States, and because many elderly people are sick and/or handicapped (and therefore incapacitated in fire situations). Fires in health care facilities are most often caused by smoking materials or suspicious acts. The article gives several charts of statistics illustrating the rates and risks for fire deaths in this population. The author suggests that compliance with the Life Safety Code, improved smoking controls, and adequate fire detection and suppression systems may help reduce the risk of fire deaths in this population.

147   *Human behavior in fire* [videotape]. (1993). Crofton, MD: Bonnie Walker & Associates, Inc.

This ten-minute video presents information on the ways people behave in fire emergencies.

148   Karter, Michael J., Jr. (February, 1992). *Patterns of fire casualties in home fires by age and sex, 1985-89.* Quincy, MA: National Fire Protection Association.

This report examines civilian casualties in homes for patterns by age and gender of victim, and looks at age and gender differences associated with various circumstances surrounding the casualty, such as the cause of the fire and the activity of the victim at time of the injury. Research indicates that preschool children under five and the elderly (ages 65 and over) have the highest rates of fire deaths in the United States. For the elderly, the rates increase dramatically with age, and the most common causes are smoking materials and heating. The author concludes that fire safety and education programs need to target these high-risk groups.

149   Karter, Michael J., Jr. (March, 1986). Patterns of fire deaths among the elderly and children in the home. *Fire Journal, 80*(3), 19-22.

The author uses statistics on fire deaths to illustrate the risk factors for young children and the elderly, and makes four conclusions: 1. that the young and very old have a much higher risk of dying in a home fire; 2. that young and very old victims of fatal fires are more likely to have limited mobility prior to the fire; 3. that young children are most often victims of fires they started themselves by playing with fire or arson; and 4. that the elderly are most often victims of fires caused by heating and cooking equipment or smoking materials.

150   Katcher, Murray L. (1992). Efforts to prevent burns from hot tap water. In Abraham B. Bergman (Ed.), *Political approaches to injury control at the state level* (pp. 69-78). Seattle, WA: University of Washington Press.

This chapter discusses the problem of tap water scalds among children, senior citizens, and physically impaired people. A 10-year retrospective review of hot tap water scalds in these high-risk groups showed that 17% were children under five, 3% were ages 65 and over, and 10% were physically or mentally disabled. The author also describes a public prevention education program which encouraged the testing and lowering of unsafe water heater temperatures in Wisconsin.

151 Katcher, Murray L., & Delventhal, Stephen J. (February, 1982). Burn injuries in Wisconsin: Epidemiology and prevention. *Wisconsin Medical Journal, 81*(2), 25-28.

A two-year study of patients admitted to the University of Wisconsin Hospital Burn Center showed that gasoline fires involving a motor vehicle or the use of gasoline to start a fire were responsible for 39% of flame burns. Flammable gases were involved in 21% of the flame burns, the most common cause was lighting a pilot light. House fires accounted for 21% of the flame burns. The majority of the electrical burns resulted from contact with a high voltage wire. Chemical burns were caused by contact with cement, fertilizers, and ammonia. Other sources of burn injury were from a heating pad, hot wood stove, hot iron casting, space heater, exhaust pipe, a drive belt (friction burn), and smoke inhalation without burns. Of the 18 fatal burns, 12 were flame burns; four were scalds (three of which were from hot tap water and occurring in the bathtub), and two were from house fires. Children under five were most commonly burned from hot liquids; two of the four cases resulted from hot tap water scalds in the bathtub.

152 Katcher, Murray L. (September, 1987). Prevention of tap water scald burns: Evaluation of a multi-media injury control program. *American Journal of Public Health, 77*(9), 1195-1197.

This prospective study evaluated the success of a tap water scald prevention program. The program included pamphlets sent through the mail, posters at doctors' offices and hospitals, and free brochures and thermometers, as well as television, radio, and newspaper announcements, and reached approximately two million people in Wisconsin. Findings indicated that the program increased the tap water scald danger awareness in the general population from 72% to 89%. However, there was no indication of any increase in the testing or lowering of water heater temperatures in this group. A sample of those who requested free thermometers showed a higher rate of testing than the general population, with 43% reporting dangerous water heater temperatures. The author suggests that a safety education program that changes awareness of risks will not necessarily change the at-risk situation or behavior, but that programs demonstrating the desired changes in behavior are more likely to prove effective.

153   Katcher, Murray L., & Shapiro, Mary Melvin. (1987). Lower
       extremity burns related to sensory loss in diabetes mellitus.
       Journal of Family Practice, 24(2), 149-151.
          The authors reviewed the cases of 37 hospitalized patients
       with diabetes mellitus who received burn therapy. The patients'
       charts revealed that 10 (27%) had suffered lower extremity burns
       related to sensory loss, most of which were caused by heat applied
       for self-treatment, usually hot tap water, moist compress, or
       heating pad. The poor circulation that accompanies diabetes
       mellitus often causes patients to use hot water or heating pads to
       diminish feelings of cold, but sensory loss often impairs the ability
       to sense when the water or heating device is too hot. The author
       suggests that physicians warn diabetes mellitus patients about the
       danger of burns during self-treatment and give recommendations
       of safe ways to warm cold feet.

154   Kirby, Randolph E. (1989). *Shenandoah Retirement Home Fire:
       Roanoke County, Virginia.* Washington, DC: Federal Emergency
       Management Agency.
          This report describes a fire at a Virginia retirement home
       that caused four deaths due to smoke inhalation. The cause was
       determined to be electrical overload that ignited paneling. In
       addition to the four fatalities, ten residents, two firefighters, and
       four police officers were injured. The report gives a detailed
       summary of the fire, as well as the building conditions that
       contributed to the fire.

155   *Leadership in public fire safety education: The year 2000 and
       beyond.* (June, 1993). Washington, DC: Federal Emergency
       Management Agency.
          This book is the result of a United States Fire Administration
       symposium to identify trends in fire prevention and safety
       education. This report identifies trends in society, in schools, in
       local government, in the fire service, and in the field of injury
       prevention and health. Based on analysis of the implications of
       these trends for public fire safety education, the book details
       future-oriented strategies and actions to maximize the impact of
       education on the nation's fire problem.

156   Levin, Bernard M., & Nelson, Harold E. (September, 1981).
       Firesafety and disabled persons. *Fire Journal, 75*(9), 35-40.
          The authors discuss the unique fire safety needs of disabled
       people. Safety regulations for the general population should be the

foundation for fire safety programs for the disabled. In addition to these general regulations, measures directly related to the individual's environment and disability should be added. The authors describe practical fire prevention techniques for these special populations, and suggest that such measures be implemented, and that the disabled people should be taught to take advantage of them.

157   Lewis, Jan. (April, 1992). Scalding tap water. *Trial, 28*(4), 74-78.
        This article describes the dangers of very hot tap water in various high-risk populations. In 1988, 5,000 United States children were scalded by hot tap water, most often in the bathroom. More than half of all fatal tap water scalds are sustained by people ages 75 and over. The very young, the very old, and the neurologically or mentally impaired may not react as quickly to hot water, and may also lack the mental ability to escape the hazard. Children and elderly people also have thinner skin and will suffer more severe burns during shorter periods of exposure than other groups. The author discusses anti-scald devices, the Safe Kids Campaign, code requirements, and court cases about scalds.

158   MacArthur, John D., & Moore, Francis D. (January 20, 1975). Epidemiology of burns: The burn-prone patient. *Journal of the American Medical Association, 231*(3), 259-263.
        The authors investigated risk factors for burns by examination of the patient history, by conversation with the family, or by physical examination of 155 adults hospitalized for burns. Factors that decreased the patient's ability to respond appropriately were considered risks. Approximately 50% of the entire sample showed predisposition to burns. Among patients with more severe burns, the proportion was 57%. Among women, predisposition was more prominent in all categories than among men. Among women, those predisposed to burning had larger burns and a greater likelihood of dying. Alcoholism led the list of predisposing factors, with senility, psychiatric disorders, and neurological disease following in order. The patient's own home was usually the site of the burn, with the initial ignition being in the patient's hair or clothing, the mattress, bedclothes, or an overstuffed chair.

159   MacKay, Annette, Halpern, Judith, McLoughlin, Elizabeth, Locke, John, & Crawford, John D. (November, 1979). A comparison of age-specific burn injury rates in five

Massachusetts communities. *American Journal of Public Health,* 69(11), 1146-1150.

The authors measured burn incidence rates for residents of five Massachusetts cities by examining all non-occupational burn injuries and cases of smoke inhalation requiring treatment on an inpatient or outpatient basis in a hospital during a three-year period. The patterns of burn injuries were similar for all five cities, indicating that different types of burn injuries correlate with certain age groups consistently. If these findings can be generalized to other geographic areas, the authors suggest that there may be behavioral or developmental factors that predispose certain age groups to certain types of burns, and that these factors may subsequently be used to form the basis for prevention efforts directed at these risk groups.

160   McLoughlin, Elizabeth & Crawford, John D. (February, 1985). Burns. *Pediatric Clinics of North America, 32*(1), 61-75.

This article discusses the six categories of burn injuries: flame, scald, contact, electrical, chemical, and ultraviolet radiation. Burns may be the result of playing with matches, smoking cigarettes, tap water scalds, kitchen scalds, or electrical cords. The article also includes information on smoke detectors, residential sprinklers, adult supervision, clothing ignition. Because the elderly and young children share high rates of burns and fire deaths, similar prevention interventions may apply to both groups.

161   Miller, Allison. (January-February, 1991). Where there's smoking there's fire. *NFPA Journal, 85*(1), 92-93.

Statistics from 1988 showed that 25% of civilian fire deaths were traced to fires caused by smoking materials. The risk of death or injury from these fires increases consistently with age. Previous attempts to prevent these fires has focused on the ignited material (such as mattresses and upholstery). The author suggests that smoking material-related fires cannot be reduced further without modifying the smoking materials or reducing the use of these materials by smokers.

162   NAHB National Research Center. (March, 1990). *Reducing fire-related injury and death among the elderly.* Upper Marlboro, MD: NAHB National Research Center.

This report provides statistical research on causes of fire in the homes of older people and the most common scenarios involving elderly people and fire. The report discusses the major types of fires and their causes: smoke, cooking equipment, heating, electrical wiring, and appliances. The authors also describe a model public education fire safety campaign for older people. The appendices include a brochure and checklist developed by project staff, materials sent to Home Builders' Associations, and materials sent to Area Agencies on Aging.

163   National Commission on Fire Prevention and Control. (1989). *America burning.* Washington, DC: U. S. Fire Administration.

This report summarizes the findings and recommendations of the National Commission on Fire Prevention and Control concerning the fire problem in the United States. The report gives statistical data about fire injuries and deaths, as well as the hazards and existing prevention efforts. The Commission recommends that an organization called the United States Fire Administration be established to meet several fire safety and prevention needs in conjunction with local governments: more emphasis on fire prevention, better training and education for fire services, fire safety education for the general public, reduced hazards in the home and workplace, improved building fire protection, and more research on firefighting and fire hazards. The United States Fire Administration would also develop a national fire data system to aid research, monitor and encourage fire research, provide fire-related bloc grants to local governments, establish a national fire academy, and coordinate a national fire safety education program.

164   Petraglia, John S. (March-April, 1991). Fire and the aging of America. *NFPA Journal, 85*(2), 37-46.

This article describes the elderly as an at-risk population for fire-related deaths and injuries. Most elderly burns and fire deaths are caused by careless use of smoking materials, alternative sources of heat, and clothing ignited while cooking. The elderly are often at higher risk than other populations because chronic medical conditions, limited mobility, and the physical effects of aging make them more vulnerable to smoke inhalation and more likely unable to escape. The author suggests that education programs, smoke detectors, and housing or furnishing designed to reduce fire risk may all help decrease the risk of fire-related injury or death among the elderly.

165   Rossomando, Christina, & Schaenman, Philip. (December, 1993). *The community-based fire safety program: Preliminary report.* Washington, DC: Tobacco Institute.

This report describes a program to distribute fire safety education literature and smoke detectors to at-risk populations at a community level. The program was originally developed in Oregon, and pilot-tested in Illinois, Maryland, and South Carolina. The program analyzed fire data in each city to identify high-risk groups and locations to determine the target group. Market research and community groups were used to plan and implement the program. Preliminary findings indicate that these pilot programs were useful in reducing fire deaths in target areas. As a result of the pilot programs, the authors developed a model program that can be used in any community to educate the public about fire safety and smoke detectors, with special emphasis on those at greatest risk from fire.

166   Schaenman, Philip, Lundquist, Barbara, Stambaugh, Hollis, Camozzo, Elyse, & Granito, Anthony. (1987). *Overcoming barriers to public fire education in the United States.* Arlington, VA: TriData.

The authors suggest that public fire education is a vital but often neglected part of fire prevention in the United States. Four groups are key players in public fire education: mayors and city managers, schools, fire services, and the insurance industry. This report outlines the barriers and problems that hinder each of these groups, and gives recommendations to improve the quality and effectiveness of current fire safety education programs.

167   Shingleton, Bradford J. (August 8, 1991). Eye injuries. *The New England Journal of Medicine, 325*(6), 408-413.

The author discusses the evaluation and prevention of eye injuries. He discusses vision threatening injuries such as chemical burns, ruptured globe (corneal laceration), and hyphema (bleeding in the anterior chamber usually resulting from blunt trauma to the globe). The home was the site of injury in 25% of patients. Children had a small proportion of the injuries overall, but a disproportionate burden of the severe injuries. Shingleton recommends wearing eye protection such as goggles or helmets with face masks.

168   Stambaugh, Hollis. (December 16, 1989). *Success story at retirement home fire: Sterling, Virginia.* Washington, DC: Federal Emergency Management Agency.

This report describes a fire incident at a Virginia retirement home. The fire started in a furnace room, and eventually spread to a contained space between the second and third floors of the building. The author attributes the lack of panic, injuries, and deaths to frequent fire drills, staff trained in emergency procedures, and the center's ambulatory population. The facility was also adequately equipped with smoke detectors, automatic alarms, and a sprinkler system.

169   Walker, Bonnie L. (July 26, 1994). *Effects of a burn prevention program on caregivers to the elderly.* Crofton, MD: Bonnie Walker & Associates.

The purpose of this study was to investigate the effects of a burn prevention program on caregivers to the elderly in nursing homes, a life care community, adult foster care homes, and the community. Caregivers completed a one-hour workshop which included a coursebook, instructor presentation and a video. Pre- and posttest data measured effects of the training on knowledge, attitudes, and planned practices. For each measured variable, the difference between pre- and posttest scores were statistically significant.

170   Walker, Bonnie L. (1993). *Fire safety in nursing facilities.* Crofton, MD: Bonnie Walker & Associates.

This coursebook provides training for staff of long-term care facilities for the elderly that practice the defend-in-place strategy in fire emergencies. Topics include the need for fire safety, human factors, fire hazards, fire emergency planning, and safety devices.

171   Walker, Bonnie L. (1990). *The fire safety workshop.* Crofton, MD: Bonnie Walker & Associates.

This coursebook is part of a training program for operators and staff of residential care facilities, group homes, and other personal care facilities for special populations. The author illustrates the need for fire safety and gives practical fire and burn prevention interventions based on how fires start and spread, the Life Safety Code, the human factors involved in awareness of and escape from fires, and the most common fire hazards. The book also includes information about the proper use and installation of fire safety devices (such as smoke detectors, sprinkler systems, emergency lights, and equipment for special populations) and ways to design and implement fire emergency plans.

172   Walker, Bonnie L. (1994). *Injury prevention for the elderly: Preventing burns and scalds.* Crofton, MD: Bonnie Walker & Associates, Inc.

This booklet was developed for caregivers of elderly people in residential care and nursing facilities. It includes information on the prevalence of burn injuries, factors which put elderly people at risk for burn injuries, and common hazards. The author also includes suggestions for prevention interventions for each common hazard.

173   Walker, Bonnie L., Beck, Kenneth, Walker, April L., & Shemanski, Susan. (May, 1992). The short-term effects of a fire safety education program for the elderly. *Fire Technology, 28*(2), 134-162.

This study evaluated a fire safety education program for the operators and staff of health care facilities and board and care homes, as well as community-dwelling elderly. The short-term effects of this training were assessed by using pre- and posttests measuring the participants' fire safety knowledge, attitudes, and practice intentions. The training was well-accepted by the participants, and the improvement in fire safety knowledge was small (8% to 10%), but significant. The findings indicate that, with some modification, a similar system of fire safety education is ready to be tested on a national level. The authors suggest that further research also measure long-term effects, specifically in the participants' behaviors.

174   Warmer weather sparks more burns. (May, 1992). *USA Today Magazine, 120*(2564), 6.

This article discusses the types of burns that are frequently seen during the summer months. Each year, more than 2,000,000 people are victims of burn injuries and between 8,000 and 12,000 die. Common causes of burns during the spring and summer include careless use of fireworks, walking barefoot on hot campfire coals, scalds from home canning, and careless use of gasoline. Approximately 75% of all burns result from the victim's own actions. Children under five and older adults are at the greatest risk for burn-related injuries and death. The article offers tips to prevent these types of burn injuries.

175   Wayside inn boarding house fire. (November, 1979). *Fire Journal, 73*(11), 28-34.

This article describes a fire at a Missouri boarding house. The fire safety requirements stipulated that a boarding house must conform to the fire, housing, and general sanitation regulations, as well as the zoning classifications of the location. In this case, there were no regulations in effect because the facility was located in unincorporated county area, and there were no state requirements. Residents were ages 24 to 96, and came from placement through the Veterans Administration, a state mental hospital, or by their own choice. All of the residents were ambulatory, and there were no wheelchairs or walkers in use at the facility. There had been no staff fire emergency training, and no fire drills for residents. Of the 37 residents and 1 attendant, 13 survived the fire, and 25 died. Some of the victims were fully or partially clothed, indicating that they had stopped to dress after discovering the fire. The nature of the building, the lack of a complete fire detection system, and the lack of emergency planning or training were the three factors associated with the high number of deaths. The article also describes the Life Safety Code requirements for similar facilities.

176   Weaver, Alissa M., Himel, Harvey N., & Edlich, Richard F. (July-August, 1993). Immersion scald burns: Strategies for prevention. *Journal of Emergency Medicine, 11*(4), 397-402.

This case study reports an elderly woman with a physical and neurological handicap who suffered scald burns covering 20% of her total body surface area while bathing. This life-threatening injury could have been prevented with a temperature-controlling water valve.

4

Choking and Asphyxiation

For people ages 90 and over, suffocation by ingestion (choking) is the second leading cause of accidental death. Elderly injuries and deaths from choking are most often due to chewing or swallowing difficulties. Conditions that contribute to choking include poor dental health, dysphagia (difficulty swallowing), achalasia (impaired ability to move matter down the esophagus), and aspiration (inhalation of matter into the airway below the pharynx). These disorders occur in all age groups, but the elderly are at higher risk for morbidity and mortality from these conditions because of multiple medical conditions, multiple medications, and age-related changes in chewing and swallowing physiology. This chapter contains journal articles that provide information on prevalence, risk factors, and environmental hazards. Some of these articles offer suggestions for practical interventions and clinical treatments that may prevent these types of injuries.

177   Atkinson, Jane C., & Fox, Philip C. (August, 1992). Salivary gland dysfunction. *Clinics in Geriatric Medicine, 8*(3), 499-512.

This article discusses the declined salivary gland function often seen in elderly patients. Salivary gland atrophy and diminished levels of saliva are not necessarily due to aging, but are more likely caused by diseases (such as Sjögren's syndrome), medications, radiation treatment, tumors, infection, alcoholic cirrhosis, and other conditions often seen in elderly patients. Patients with decreased levels of saliva for any of these reasons should use salivary stimulants such as gum or lemon drops, avoid caffeinated beverages that may cause dehydration, use humidifiers at home, and avoid foods that can irritate unlubricated mouths and throats.

178   Bird, Margaret R., Woodward, Michael C., Gibson, Elizabeth M., Phyland, Debra J., & Fonda, David. (May, 1994). Asymptomatic swallowing disorders in elderly patients with Parkinson's disease: A description of findings on clinical examination and videofluoroscopy in sixteen patients. *Age and Ageing, 23*(3), 251-254.

This Australian study examined 16 elderly men and women (ages 65 and over) with Parkinson's disease. The subjects were assessed by self-report questionnaire for symptoms of dysphagia (difficulty swallowing), and were found to have no symptoms. Swallowing tests showed that all 16 subjects showed at least one abnormality. Three subjects showed aspiration while swallowing, and 14 showed vallecular residue, a symptom considered a risk factor for aspiration. The authors suggest that self-reports of swallowing in Parkinson's patients may not be reliable, and that these patients may be at risk for aspiration, even when symptoms of swallowing difficulties or choking are not present. Because aspiration while swallowing is a significant contributor to morbidity and mortality in this population, complete assessment of swallowing difficulty is essential.

179   Castell, Donald O. (June, 1990). Esophageal disorders in the elderly. *Gastroenterology Clinics of North America, 19*(2), 235-254.

This article describes esophageal disorders common to the elderly. The three most common symptoms of these disorders are dysphagia (difficulty swallowing), chest pains, and heartburn. There are two types of dysphagia: oropharyngeal, which affects the muscles controlling the tongue, pharynx, and upper sphincter; and esophageal, which affects the esophagus itself. Oropharyngeal dysphagia in the elderly is often the result of cerebrovascular accidents (major strokes, Wallenberg's syndrome), neuromuscular disorders (Parkinson's disease, polymyositis, myasthenia gravis, thyroid problems), tumors, and other disorders. Esophageal dysphagia may be caused by muscular disorders or obstructions, and may create symptoms of chest pains. Gastroesophageal reflux may cause heartburn. Treatment of these conditions in the elderly are similar to those used in younger patients, but clinicians should be aware of the elderly's greater risk of drug interactions when prescribing treatment.

180 *Choking: To save a life* [videotape]. (1989). Chicago, IL: Encyclopaedia Britannica Educational Corporation.

This 12-minute video demonstrates choking rescue techniques such as the Heimlich maneuver and the finger probe.

181 Day, Richard L., Crelin, Edmund S., & DuBois, Arthur B. (July, 1982). Choking: The Heimlich abdominal thrust vs back blows: An approach to measurement of inertial and aerodynamic forces. *Pediatrics, 70*(1), 113-119.

The authors tested the effectiveness of back blows as compared to the Heimlich maneuver in first-aid for infant and adult choking. The back blows produced less pressure than the Heimlich thrusts when subjects were seated, and were more likely to cause foreign matter to drop further down and backward, rather than up and out. The Heimlich maneuver, then, is the more effective method of handling choking with the least risk of making partial blockage into complete obstruction.

182 Eisele, David W. (1991). Surgical approaches to aspiration. *Dysphagia, 6*(2), 71-78.

Aspiration occurs when secretions, oral intake, or gastric contents penetrate the larynx and enter the airway below the vocal cords. This condition can cause a series of disorders, including pneumonia, bronchitis, and other bronchopulmonary problems. Depending on the nature and amount of aspirated material, the patient may also be at risk for choking or suffocation. The author describes various treatments for this disorder.

183 Ergun, Gulchin A., & Miskovitz, Paul F. (1992). Aging and the esophagus: Common pathologic conditions and their effect upon swallowing in the geriatric population. *Dysphagia, 7*(2), 58-63.

Dysphagia (difficulty swallowing) is not necessarily a function of age; however, age-related changes and chronic problems may exacerbate pre-existing swallowing problems. Esophageal dysphagia refers to difficulties passing food through the esophagus. This may be caused by muscular disorders, which decrease the ability to move food through the esophagus, or by injuries or lesions that block the esophagus. Gastroesophageal reflux disease occurs when stomach contents escape into the esophagus, and may be exacerbated by many medications, hormones, and foods. In severely dysphagic elder patients, swallowing processes must be evaluated and treated to prevent choking and malnutrition.

184   **Feinberg, Michael J. (Fall, 1993). Radiographic techniques and interpretation of abnormal swallowing in adult and elderly patients.** *Dysphagia, 8*(4), 356-358.

This article describes the basic components of swallowing to illustrate the nature and stages of various swallowing problems. The author also discusses current techniques of swallowing assessment, including videofluoroscopy.

185   **Feinberg, Michael J., Knebl, Janice, Tully, Joann, & Segall, Linda. (1990). Aspiration and the elderly.** *Dysphagia, 5*(2), 61-71.

This article is a review of aspiration, a condition where food or other matter enters the airway beyond the larynx. In elderly people, aspiration is a prevalent problem. The consequences of this condition depend on the matter swallowed, the amount swallowed, and the patient's health, but may include aspiration pneumonia, pulmonary disease, food asphyxia, coughing, and potentially fatal choking. The authors suggest that aging causes the sensitivity of the larynx to decrease, allowing foreign matter to pass through. Difficulty eating because of aspiration may also lead to vomiting, fear of eating, and malnutrition. Diagnosis of aspiration involves videofluoroscopy, which uses swallowed barium to measure amounts of matter aspirated. For patients with this condition, management often includes eliminating thin liquids, such as water, coffee, or tea, while monitoring ingestion of solid or semi-solid foods to prevent choking. Other treatment options include surgical measures and tube feeding.

186   **Galindo-Ciocon, Daisy J. (June, 1993). Tube feeding: Complications among the elderly.** *Journal of Gerontological Nursing, 19*(6), 17-22.

The author describes the various complications associated with tube feeding in elderly patients. These complications include diarrhea, aspiration, agitation, clogging, and patient complaints. The author describes each complication with its possible causes, and gives recommendations to prevent these problems. Proper use of tube feeding in conjunction with these recommended prevention interventions may enable the nurse to provide safe and effective nutrition for elderly patients who must be tube fed.

187 Gorman, Robert C., Morris, Jon B., & Kaiser, Larry R. (February, 1994). Esophageal disease and the elderly patient. *Surgical Clinics of North America, 74*(1), 93-112.

The authors describe esophageal disorders among the elderly. These disorders are often manifested in dysphagia (difficulty swallowing), regurgitation, chest pain, and heartburn. Diagnosis of these disorders is often difficult because the symptoms are often attributable to underlying cardiac and pulmonary disease. The elderly are more susceptible to the subsequent complications of these disorders, which may include aspiration and malnutrition. The authors suggest that, due to increased risk of complications, esophageal disorders in elderly patients must be detected early, and treated quickly.

188 Hogstel, Mildred O., & Robinson, Nell B. (March, 1989). Feeding the frail elderly. *Journal of Gerontological Nursing, 15*(3), 16-20.

This article gives practical solutions for nurse aides who are responsible for monitoring and feeding frail elderly residents. By understanding the types of foods that are likely to cause choking, aspiration, or other physical and dietary problems in this population, nursing facility staff can provide a diet that is both safe and nutritionally adequate. The article includes diagrams of suggested place settings and feeding areas, as well as sample diets.

189 Hotaling, Denise L. (1992). Nutritional considerations for the pureed diet texture in dysphagic elderly. *Dysphagia, 7*(2), 81-85.

Because an estimated 15% to 20% of patients in long-term care need pureed diets to compensate for difficulties chewing, digesting, or swallowing, the author describes the methods and techniques that can make pureed diets appealing and nutritionally adequate. If these diets are both adequate and flavorful, the implications of "baby food" are reduced, patient compliance may improve, and the experience may prove more enjoyable for both staff and residents. The article also includes several sample recipes.

190 Khawaja, Imran T., Buffa, Salvatore D., & Brandstetter, Robert D. (July, 1992). Aspiration pneumonia: A threat when deglutition is compromised. *Postgraduate Medicine, 92*(1), 165-181.

This article reviews aspiration pneumonia, a condition that often occurs as a result of aspiration of food or other matter. Risk factors for this condition include increased age, a change in mental status, difficult deglutition (swallowing), gastroesophageal reflux, alcoholism, seizures, cerebrovascular accident, anesthesia, tube feeding, drug addiction, and other disorders. Complications may include recurring aspiration, fever, respiratory problems, pneumonia, and death from asphyxiation. Aspiration and swallowing disorders occur in all age groups, but the elderly are particularly at risk because of increased prevalence and greater morbidity and mortality as a result of dietary problems. Current treatment focuses on supportive care, and the treatment of resulting complications.

191   Kikuchi, Ryo, Watabe, Nobuyuki, Konno, Tamohiko, Mishina, Naoko, Sekizawa, Kiyohisa, & Sasaki, Hidetada. (1994). High incidence of silent aspiration in elderly patients with community-acquired pneumonia. *American Journal of Respiratory and Critical Care Medicine, 150*(1), 251-253.

This study examined 14 elderly patients (ages 63 and over) admitted to a Japanese hospital for community-acquired pneumonia and 10 age-matched control subjects. Findings indicated that 71% of the patients aspirated, compared to 10% of control subjects. The authors suggest that elderly people frequently aspirate, and that aspiration pneumonia may occur in these situations because normal pulmonary defenses are impaired.

192   Logemann, Jeri A. (1993). Noninvasive approaches to deglutitive aspiration. *Dysphagia, 8*(4), 331-333.

Deglutitive aspiration occurs when food or other matter penetrates the vocal folds and enters the airway. Normal response to this type of penetration would be a cough to clear the material. In patients with dysphagia, there is often no cough response. This condition is referred to as silent aspiration. Management of aspiration involves identifying and treating the physiological cause, often by changing posture while swallowing, using different swallowing techniques, increasing oral sensation, or performing exercises to improve swallowing mechanisms.

193   Logemann, Jeri A. (December, 1990). Effects of aging on the swallowing mechanism. *Otolaryngologic Clinics of North America, 23*(6), 1045-1056.

The author describes swallowing, which normally involves fine neuromuscular control. Aging may affect this process in three ways: primary effects, which occur as a result of aging itself; secondary effects, which are a result of chronic medical conditions commonly suffered by the elderly; and tertiary, which are related to the environmental, social, and psychological factors of aging.

Primary effects include an increase in some tissues in the tongue and a reduction in the ability to chew and/or swallow. Medications, neurologic damage (from stroke, Parkinson's disease, dementia, or other damage), arthritis, head or neck cancer, and the general weakness associated with illness and reduced mobility can all create secondary effects on the swallowing mechanism. The author suggests that any older adult complaining of swallowing problems should receive a complete swallowing assessment and treatment because the elderly are at particular risk for serious complications such as choking or impaired nutritional intake.

194 Martin, K. Udell, & Martin, J. O'Hara. (1992). Meeting the oral health needs of institutionalized elderly. *Dysphagia, 7*(2), 73-80.
This article is an overview of dental and oral health for institutionalized elderly people. Because poor dental health can contribute to choking or malnutrition, the use of special dentures may improve the patients' ability to chew food, and subsequently ease swallowing. The authors describe and recommend several other tools and techniques for the prevention of further dental decay, the treatment of swallowing problems, the identification of oral and dental problems, and the preservation of patients' independence by maintaining their own oral health.

195 Mendez, Leonardo, Friedman, Lawrence S., & Castell, Donald O. (May, 1991). Swallowing disorders in the elderly. *Clinics in Geriatric Medicine, 7*(2), 215-230.
The authors review the oropharyngeal and esophageal disorders most common in the elderly. Symptoms of dysphagia, heartburn, and chest pain are the presenting manifestations of these disorders in all ages, but these symptoms in an elderly patient may be clouded by other chronic conditions. The elderly suffer from many of the same esophageal disorders as younger people; however, some disorders are unique to the elderly, and the frequency of some disorders increases with age. The treatment of these disorders is similar to that used for younger patients, but clinicians should be cautious when prescribing medication, because the elderly are at increased risk for adverse drug reactions and interactions.

196 Oppenheimer, Stephen, & Hachinski, Vladimir. (March 21, 1992). Complications of acute stroke. *Lancet, 339*(8795), 721-725.
The authors describe the aftermath of an acute stroke. Because the rate of fatality from stroke and/or stroke

complications is high, recognition of complications is vital to the treatment of stroke victims. The most common cause of death following a stroke is transtentorial herniation, which is a disorder caused by increased pressure in the brain. Other complications include brain hemorrhage, seizures, depression, endocrine imbalances, high blood pressure, fever, infection, pressure sores, blood clots, dysphagia, silent aspiration, and coronary problems. Stroke therapy involving several medications may also cause complications such as sedation or depression, adverse drug reactions, hormonal imbalances, and hemorrhage.

197   Riley, Mary Ellen, & Volicer, Ladislav. (March, 1990). Evaluation of a new nutritional supplement for patients with Alzheimer's disease. *Journal of the American Dietetic Association, 90*(3), 433-436.

      The authors tested a nutritional supplement for elderly Alzheimer's patients. Because Alzheimer's disease causes eating problems such as holding food in the mouth and forgetting how to eat or swallow, nutritional supplements are often necessary. Subjects were 13 patients who had been classified as difficult to feed as a result of a history of choking on liquids or solids, failing to adequately chew before swallowing, and other eating problems. Eight of the patients received the study supplement for 35 days, and then received other commonly used supplements for 35 days. The process was reversed for the other five subjects. Despite the fact that feeding problems were still encountered during the study, the study supplement was shown to decrease choking in one patient, and to take less feeding time among all subjects. The authors suggest that the feeding complications of Alzheimer's disease necessitate careful evaluation of nutrition and nutritional supplements to reduce the risk of malnutrition, choking, aspiration, and asphyxiation.

198   Rund, Douglas A. (December, 1989). Airway obstruction: The Heimlich maneuver. *The Physician and Sportsmedicine, 17*(12), 36-39.

      This article gives an overview of the history and mechanics of the Heimlich maneuver. Tests on animal and human subjects have shown this technique effective in preventing deaths and serious injuries from choking on food. If performed correctly, the Heimlich maneuver can be used by a minimally trained person to safely dislodge food or other material obstructing the choking victim's airway. The author uses illustrations to demonstrate this technique, and gives instructions for various choking situations.

199   Sonies, Barbara C. (August, 1992). **Oropharyngeal dysphagia in the elderly.** *Clinics in Geriatric Medicine, 8*(3), 569-577.

   This article discusses the swallowing problems that elderly people often experience. Although aging may affect the physical mechanisms that control swallowing, dysphagia is more often due to disease or medications that are more common in the elderly. Elderly suffering from swallowing disorders are more often institutionalized in an effort to maintain their nutritional health, but this maintenance (usually in the form of tube feeding and/or nutritional supplements) has its own set of complications (aspiration, infection, or bleeding) and a range of ethical problems for caregivers.

200   Sonies, Barbara C., & Dalakas, Marinos C. (April 25, 1991). **Dysphagia in patients with the post-polio syndrome.** *New England Journal of Medicine, 324*(17), 1162-1168.

   This study assessed the risk of swallowing problems after an attack of acute paralytic poliomyelitis. Subjects were 32 patients with post-polio syndrome, defined here by new weakness in the arms and legs. Of these 32 subjects, 14 had symptoms of new swallowing problems, and 18 had no symptoms. Twelve subjects had a history of oropharyngeal involvement in attacks of acute poliomyelitis. Swallowing tests showed that all but one of the subjects had some swallowing abnormality. The authors conclude that patients with post-polio syndrome may also have muscular dysfunction in swallowing that is similar to the muscular degeneration in the arms and legs that is typical of this disorder.

201   Tibbling, Lita, & Gustafsson, Barbro. (1991). **Dysphagia and its consequences in the elderly.** *Dysphagia, 6*(4), 200-202.

   This Swedish study analyzed the frequency and related symptoms of dysphagia in community-dwelling elderly (ages 60 and over). Subjects were 796 elderly residents of a Swedish city; 46% were men, 60% were ages 60 to 69, 29% were ages 70 to 79, and 7% were ages 80 and over. Sixty-two (8%) of the subjects had symptoms of dysphagia. These subjects were more likely to suffer from chest pain, heartburn, regurgitation, and a history of heart problems than the other subjects. The authors conclude that elderly people with dysphagia also suffer from physical and psychosocial complications that are either not recognized or not properly treated by doctors, resulting in a reduced quality of life for this population.

202   **Williams, Janet M., & Evans, Timothy C. (August, 1993). Acute pulmonary disease in the aged.** *Clinics in Geriatric Medicine,* *9*(3), 527-546.

This article reviews the most common non-infectious pulmonary emergencies among the elderly. Pulmonary embolism, which occurs when the artery to the lungs becomes clogged, is often fatal, and the elderly are at particular risk for this problem because of pre-existing cardiac and pulmonary disease. Lung diseases such as asthma, chronic bronchitis, and emphysema can put the elderly at risk for asphyxiation and obstructed breathing. Aspiration can be a significant risk of morbidity and mortality for the elderly because of decreased gag and cough reflexes. Adult respiratory distress syndrome and lung cancer are other sources of high mortality rates in the elderly. The authors suggest that age-related physiological changes in respiratory mechanisms, in conjunction with medical conditions and medication complications, can make the elderly less tolerant of these respiratory disorders, and at higher risk of death or serious injury from respiratory problems.

203   **Zikk, Daniel, Rapoport, Yoram, Papo, Joseph, Halperin, Doron, & Himelfarb, Mordechai Z. (August, 1989). Acute airway obstruction and achalasia of the esophagus.** *Annals of Otology, Rhinology, and Laryngology, 98*(8), 641-643.

Achalasia is a muscular disorder of the esophagus that impairs a person's ability to swallow food. The authors describe the case of a 74-year-old woman with a history of dysphagia and coughing admitted to the emergency room with breathing difficulty after eating. Examination revealed that she had aspirated as a result of achalasia. The authors report that achalasia-related respiratory problems, such as choking or airway obstruction, commonly follow the regurgitation and aspiration of food matter.

5

Drowning

Drowning is one of the leading causes of accidental death for people ages 65 and over. These fatalities often occur in bathtubs, but are also associated with swimming, fishing, and boating accidents. Risk factors for drowning accidents include seizure disorders, use of alcohol, and participating in activities near water. The articles included in this chapter discuss prevalence, risk factors, and environmental hazards. A few writers offer prevention suggestions such as controlling or prohibiting alcohol consumption at water sites and, for those at risk of seizures, taking showers rather than baths.

204 Budnick, Lawrence D., & Ross, David A. (June, 1985). Bathtub-related drownings in the United States, 1979-81. *American Journal of Public Health, 75*(6), 630-633.

This study used National Center for Health Statistics and Consumer Product Safety Commission data to evaluate bathtub-related drownings and injuries in the United States from 1979 to 1981. During 1979 to 1980, 710 people drowned in bathtubs. Rates were lowest in New England and highest in Pacific and Mountain states. Young children and the elderly were at the highest risk. Personal risk factors varied with age and included a history of being left unattended (for children under five), frequent history of seizures (ages 5 to 39), history of alcohol or drug use (ages 40 to 59), and a history of falls (ages 60 and over). In addition to eliminating personal risks, modifying bathrooms to counteract slippery surfaces and taking showers instead of baths may decrease the risk of drowning in bathtubs for all age groups.

205   Dietz, Park E., & Baker, Susan P. (April, 1974). Drowning: Epidemiology and prevention. *American Journal of Public Health, 64*(4), 303-312.

The authors reviewed records of accidental drowning deaths in Maryland to determine their relationship to age, ethnicity, alcohol use, disease, and other factors. These deaths were in three groups: 16 deaths during Tropical Storm Agnes, 117 other deaths in 1972, and 45 adult drowning deaths in Baltimore City from 1968 to 1972. Deaths from drownings most often involved swimming (34%) and boating (29%), but rarely involved swimming in the ocean or sailing. Drowning rates were higher for males, especially those ages 15-24. Bathtub drownings were most often related to preexisting conditions, usually seizure disorders. In the Baltimore City group, 47% of drowning victims had positive blood alcohol tests. The authors suggest that prevention efforts include water safety education for high-risk groups, highly visible swimwear, and informing patients about the dangers of use of alcohol while participating in water sports.

206   Gulaid, Jama A., & Sattin, Richard W. (1988). Drownings in the United States, 1978-1984. *Morbidity and Mortality Weekly Report, 37*(SS-1), 27-33.

The authors used National Center for Health Statistics Data to determine the number of deaths by drowning in the United States from 1978 to 1984. During the seven years studied, an average of 6,503 persons drowned each year, ranging from a high of 7,026 in 1978 to a low of 5,388 in 1984. Children ages five and under and young adults between ages 15 to 24 had the highest drowning rates. The circumstances of drowning varied by age group: swimming pools were the greatest hazard for toddlers and bathtub drownings were the most common for children and adults ages 70 and over. Drowning rates vary according to climate, geographic location, and a variety of personal risk factors. The authors conclude that the drop in fatalities from 1978 to 1984 shows some progress in the prevention of drownings, but suggest that more research and prevention efforts are necessary, especially among the high-risk groups established in this study.

207   Howland, Jonathan, Mangione, Thomas, Hingson, Ralph, Levenson, Suzette, Winter, Michael, & Altwicker, Andrea. (July-

August, 1990). A pilot survey of aquatic activities and related consumption of alcohol, with implications for drowning. *Public Health Reports, 105*(4), 415-419.

This study examined the relationship between alcohol consumption and water sports. Subjects were 294 respondents (ages 20 and over) to a telephone survey, out of which 79% of men and 72% of women reported participating in aquatic activities within the past month. The most common activities were swimming, sunbathing, power boating, and fishing. Subjects who reported consuming alcohol during these activities (36% of men and 11% of women) were more likely to report having driven after drinking. The authors suggest that federal and state efforts to curb drinking and boating should include educational programs about the dangers of drinking alcohol while participating in water activities.

208 *Medical analysis of swimming pool injuries.* (December, 1977). Washington, DC: U. S. Product Safety Commission.

This report discusses a study of 72 swimming pool injuries, including the circumstances of the injuries, characteristics of the victims, and lingering results of the injuries. Only one victim in the study was aged 0-6, and three were ages 49 and over. The majority were ages 13 to 24, and 62 of the 72 victims were male. The authors use the information gained from the study to make recommendations for drowning prevention and a safer pool environment: improved pool design, better supervision, and adequate rescue and medical care.

209 Metropolitan Life Insurance Company. (May, 1977). Accidental drownings by age and activity. *Statistical Bulletin, 58*, 2-5.

This study examined 4,962 drowning fatalities to review the various activities in which drowning victims were engaged prior to death. Swimming was the most frequently mentioned activity, with 1,238 deaths (25% of all drowning deaths) attributed to such activity. Playing near bodies of water resulted in 697 deaths (14% of the total), and 343 deaths occurred while fishing from a boat (7%). Recreational boating was reported in 349 drownings. Drownings in nonrecreational situations occurred while driving a motor vehicle (355 cases), attempting a rescue (143 cases), and bathing (100 cases). Activities varied by age: children under five were susceptible to drowning while bathing, playing near water, and standing or walking near water. Children ages 5 to 14 accounted for a majority of bathing or wading as well as swimming drownings. Boating, diving, and fishing drownings were more common among ages 15 to 44. The elderly (ages 65 and over) drowned most often after walking or standing near water.

210   North Carolina drownings, 1980-1984. (October 10, 1986). *Morbidity and Mortality Weekly Report, 35*(40), 635-638.

According to medical examiner records, a total of 1,052 persons drowned in North Carolina from 1980 to 1984. Death rates were higher for nonwhites and for males. Most of the drownings occurred in natural settings such as lakes or rivers. Most victims were swimming (41%) or fishing (15%). Drowning circumstances varied by age, gender, and medical conditions. Males accounted for 98% of fishing deaths, and females accounted for 43% of bath-related deaths. Out of the 80% tested, alcohol was detected in 48% of the victims, and 34% had blood-alcohol levels equal to or above the legal level of intoxication.

211   O'Carroll, Patrick W., Alkon, Ellen, & Weiss, Billie. (July 15, 1988). Drowning mortality in Los Angeles County, 1976-1984. *Journal of the American Medical Association, 260*(3), 380-382.

The authors examined Los Angeles County Coroner's Office data on drownings from 1976 to 1984. There were 1,587 drownings (1,130 males, 457 females) during this nine-year period. The largest proportion of drownings (44.5%) for both sexes and for most age groups occurred in private swimming pools. Drowning circumstances varied by age and gender. Children ages two to three had the highest swimming pool drowning rate. The elderly also showed high drowning rates, mostly in swimming pools and bathtubs. The authors suggest that prevention interventions directed toward at-risk age groups in their individual at-risk environments (such as safety regulations governing pool fencing and bathroom safety devices for the elderly) may help reduce the number of deaths due to drowning.

212   Plueckhahn, Vernon D. (1977). Alcohol and accidental submersion from watercraft and surrounds. *Medicine, Science, and the Law, 77*(4), 246-250.

The author describes the physical mechanisms associated with drowning, and the association of alcohol consumption with drowning deaths. The author suggests that elevated blood-alcohol levels may be responsible for many drowning deaths, especially in cases where the victim does not appear to struggle or try to swim, and recommends that the public should be educated about the dangers of drinking alcohol while boating or prior to swimming.

213 Plueckhahn, Vernon D. (July 7, 1984). Alcohol and accidental drowning: A 25-year study. *The Medical Journal of Australia,* *141*(1), 22-25.

The author studied autopsy records of Australian drowning deaths from 1958 to 1983 to examine the relationship of alcohol to death by drowning. Findings showed that 37% of the male victims and 51% of victims ages 30 to 64 had a blood-alcohol level ≥.08. The physiological effects of alcohol consumption may lead to a tendency to engage in high-risk behavior and to an inability to respond, swim, or struggle after submersion. The author suggests that cautions against combining alcohol consumption with water-related activity are just as important as cautions against swimming after eating.

214 Press, Edward, Walker, James, & Crawford, Isabelle. (December, 1968). An interstate drowning study. *American Journal of Public Health, 58*(12), 2275-2289.

This study examined 1,201 drownings in five states during a 12-month period. Children and young adults ages 10 to 19 accounted for a majority of drownings. The site of drowning (pond, ocean, swimming pool) varied according to geographic location. Males accounted for a majority of deaths (84.9%), but the ratio is less significant in the very young (ages 0 to 4) and elderly (ages 65 and over). Most victims who drowned while swimming were ages 10 to 19. Ability to swim, use of life preservers, preexisting medical conditions, artificial respiration, attempts to save others, use of alcohol, and cold water affected the likelihood of death by drowning.

215 Wintemute, Garen J., Kraus, Jess F., Teret, Stephen P., & Wright, Mona A. (1988). The epidemiology of drowning in adulthood: Implications for prevention. *American Journal of Preventive Medicine, 4*(6), 343-348.

This study used Sacramento County, California drowning death records from 1974 to 1985 to discover whether the epidemiology of adult drownings is different from previous studies that focused mainly on children. The findings suggest that high-risk situations for adults are much more diverse and difficult to categorize than those for children. A majority of childhood drownings occur in swimming pools or bathtubs, and prevention efforts can be narrowed to concentrate on these risk areas. For adults, however, a variety of risk areas and risk factors necessitates a broad array of prevention efforts. The single most pervasive factor related to the drownings in this study was alcohol intoxication, which was involved in nearly half of the cases studied, suggesting that alcohol consumption should be controlled or prohibited at water sites. A history of seizures was a factor in bathtub drownings, suggesting that those at risk should take showers rather than baths. Drownings among motor vehicle occupants were nearly as common as among boaters. To prevent these deaths, the authors suggest promoting the use of seatbelts and airbags, modifying high-risk road areas, and curbing drinking and driving.

6

Elder Abuse

Elder abuse is not a class of injuries, such as drowning or choking; however, the problem is wide-spread and poses a major threat to older people. Types of abuse include physical, psychological, financial, and social abuse. Elder abuse also includes neglect. Many of the articles in this chapter attempt to describe or define elder abuse. Other writers discuss risk factors such as dementia, frailty, and abusive behavior toward caregivers. Many writers focus on the caregiver and research on the reasons for abuse and interventions. Abuse occurs in both community settings and institutions and the articles in this section discuss both environments. Elder abuse also includes crime and violence toward the elderly.

216   All, Anita C. (July, 1994). A literature review: Assessment and intervention in elder abuse. *Journal of Gerontological Nursing*, 20(7), 25-32.

The author reviews current literature on abuse of the elderly. Despite recent exposure of this problem, there are still no uniform definitions of the exact nature of elder abuse. Identification of abuse is difficult, except in cases of outright, visible battering, and is often dependent both on the setting and the health workers' or caregivers' perception of abuse. Indicators of abuse include the following: a pattern of changing health care repeatedly, missed appointments, unexplained injuries, burns in unusual locations, bruises, poor personal hygiene, sexually transmitted diseases, extreme changes in mood, depression, fearfulness, and overconcern with health care cost. The typical victim of elder abuse is female, over 75, white, living with a relative, and having some kind of physical or mental impairment. There are several existing screening instruments for elder abuse, but assessment and intervention are still difficult because of the ethical and legal issues involved. The author recommends that future studies investigate the reliability of current screening measures, as well as the complex issues still unresearched in this area.

217   Anetzberger, Georgia J., Korbin, Jill E., & Austin, Craig. (June, 1994). Alcoholism and elder abuse. *Journal of Interpersonal Violence, 9*(2), 184-193.

This comparison group study examined the relationship between caregiver alcohol use and abuse and violence against the elderly. Subjects were 23 adult children identified as abusers of their elderly parents, and 39 adult children who cared for their elderly parents, but had no reported history of abuse. Findings showed that abusers were twice as likely to have used alcohol in the past two years than the non-abusers. Of the abusers who used alcohol, 61.5% drank daily, and half of them drank three or more drinks. The authors suggest that these findings indicate that there is a significant relationship between alcoholism and elder abuse, and recommend that future research examine this relationship more specifically.

218   Ansello, Edward F., King, Nancy R., & Taler, George. (1986). The environmental press model: A theoretical framework for intervention in elder abuse. In Karl A. Pillemer, & Rosalie S. Wolf (Eds.), *Elder abuse: Conflict in the family* (pp. 314-330). Dover, MA: Auburn House Publishing Company.

This chapter explains the environmental press model for elder abuse intervention. Environmental press refers to the demands of the caregiving environment. For instance, patients who need constant supervision exact more demanding attention from the caregiver. Theoretically, the caregiver who can successfully adapt his or her personal level of competence to the environmental press will be at decreased risk for stress-related abuse and neglect. Maladaptation may occur when competence and press are out of proportion. This may happen two ways: the caregiver whose competence exceeds the environmental needs of his or her patient may be prone to boredom, which may lead to neglect; in a different way, the caregiver who is incapable of adapting to the overwhelming needs of his or her patient may become aggressive or angry toward the patient, which may lead to abuse. In this model, intervention involves stabilizing environmental press and caregiver competence. While this method may not serve all situations of abuse and neglect, the authors suggest that the model may help intervene in situations of stress-related elder abuse and neglect.

219   Benedek, Elissa P. (December, 1993). Violence: The malignancy of our times! Is there hope? *American Journal of Psychoanalysis,* 53(4), 283-293.

The author describes the increasing levels of violence in America. This violence takes many forms: homicides, spousal abuse, child abuse, elder abuse, and interpersonal violence. Three cases are described: a ten-year-old girl living with her aunt because she had been abused by her parents, a woman doctor abused by her husband, and an elderly Chinese woman abused by her son. Environmental factors that may contribute to this violence include social isolation, abuse of alcohol and drugs and easy access to weapons. Because the causes of violence are many and complex, there is no one solution to the problem of violence. The author suggests that violence prevention includes decreasing the cultural acceptance of violence in schools and in the media and raising the communities' awareness of the violence and its causes.

220   Benton, Donna, & Marshall, Charles. (November, 1991). Elder abuse. *Clinics in Geriatric Medicine,* 7(4), 831-846.

This article reviews the different types of elder abuse, which encompass physical, psychological, and financial abuse and also include the violation of personal rights, or social abuse. Detection of elder abuse can be hampered by the denial or shame of the abused and the denial or improper assessment by health care workers, or by ethical problems faced by professionals in cases of suspected abuse. Misinformation, the caregiver's lack of understanding of the needs of older adults, social isolation, a history of dysfunctional family relationships, and the psychopathologic factors of the caregiver are factors associated with elder abuse. Caregiver stress is also a factor in elder abuse situations. Self-neglect is the most commonly reported type of elder abuse, but is the most difficult to handle, because the elderly have a right to refuse services. To adequately asses elder abuse, the authors recommend examination of the following: physical indicators (bruises, malnutrition, fractures), as well as the patient's social, family, sexual, and psychological history. The caregiver's psychological history is also important. The authors also suggest that physicians and other health care workers become familiar with the reporting laws in their states.

221   Blakely, Bernard E., & Dolon, Ronald. (Winter, 1991). The relative contributions of occupation groups in the discovery and treatment of elder abuse and neglect. *Journal of Gerontological Social Work, 17*(1-2), 183-200.

To assess the effectiveness of different occupation groups in cases of elder abuse, the authors analyzed data from 334 personnel from Area Agencies on Aging in 32 states. Subjects were asked to rank the helpfulness of 14 occupational groups for abuse and neglect at both the discovery and treatment stages of intervention. The results of the survey may indicate those factors which might influence the cooperation of different occupation groups in the prevention and detection of elder abuse, and in the effectiveness of elder abuse intervention.

222   Blakely, Bernard E., Dolon, Ronald, & May, Douglas D. (1993). Improving the responses of physicians to elder abuse and neglect: Contributions of a model program. *Journal of Gerontological Social Work, 19*(3-4), 35-47.

This article describes a cooperative training-service program used by the Southeast Multi-Service Center and the Geriatric Unit of the Indiana University Department of General Internal Medicine. The program allows physicians to conduct home visits to clients who are in need of medical evaluations and services, and permits medical students to experience the elderly in home environments and the perspectives of social service providers and protective services investigators. The authors describe several elder abuse case reports to illustrate the program, and suggest that similar programs could help physicians and other professionals become familiar with the human qualities of their patients, and could also make them aware of the social service aspects of medical care and cases of abuse and neglect.

223   Carr, Kathleen, Dix, Gretchen, Fulmer, Terry, Kavesh, William, Kravitz, Liebe, Matlaw, Jane, Mayer, Jane, Minaker, Kenneth, Shapiro, Michael, Street, Shirley, Wetle, Terrie, & Zarle, Nancy. (April, 1986). An elder abuse assessment team in an acute hospital setting. *The Gerontologist, 26*(2), 115-118.

The authors describe an elder abuse assessment team at Beth Israel Hospital in Boston, Massachusetts. The Elder Assessment

Team was established in 1981 in response to a Massachusetts mandatory abuse reporting law. The team is composed of five nurses, three social workers, three physicians, and one health policy and ethics specialist. Once a suspected abused elder is referred to the team, the patient is given a preliminary assessment. If, after initial assessment, further action is deemed necessary, the team will initiate a multidisciplinary assessment. The case is then presented and evaluated for action at a weekly team meeting. The authors suggest that a multidisciplinary team will improve the accuracy and reduce the ethical implications of screening and intervention in suspected cases of elder abuse.

224 Coyne, Andrew C., Reichman, William E., & Berbig, Lisa J. (April, 1993). The relationship between dementia and elder abuse. *American Journal of Psychiatry, 150*(4), 643-646.

This study examined the relationship between dementia patients and abuse by caregivers. The research sent an anonymous questionnaire to 1,000 caregivers who called a telephone help-line specializing in dementia. Questionnaires were completed by 342 caregivers. The mean age of caregivers was 56.1 years; 163 (54.5%) were adult children caring for parents, 111 (37.1%) cared for spouses, and 25 (8.4%) cared for other relatives. Thirty-three caregivers (11.9%) reported that they had directed physically abusive behavior (such as pinching, shoving, biting, kicking, striking) toward their patient. These caregivers had been providing care for more years, were caring for patients functioning at a lower level, displayed higher burden scores, and displayed higher depression scores than caregivers who reported no abuse. In addition, 92 caregivers (33.1%) reported that the patient directed abuse toward them during the course of providing care. Caregivers who had been abused by patients, in comparison to those who had not, were more likely to direct abusive behavior back toward the patient in their care. The authors suggest that abuse involving dementia patients may be associated with the extreme psychological and physical demands placed on family members who care for relatives with dementia.

225 Daniels, R. Steven, Baumhover, Lorin A., & Clark-Daniels, Carolyn L. (1989). Physicians' mandatory reporting of elder abuse. *The Gerontologist, 29*(3), 321-327.

This study examined the effectiveness of laws mandating that physicians report cases of elder abuse. The authors surveyed licensed physicians in Alabama during the summer of 1987 to determine the physicians' knowledge of elder abuse and neglect, their understanding of the law, and their willingness to report cases of abuse and neglect. The physicians gave mixed responses to the questions. For example, over 60% believed that an experienced physician could accurately diagnose abuse; however, 77% were doubtful or uncertain about clear-cut definitions of abuse. Over one-half were unsure if their state had standard procedures for dealing with abuse, and three-fourths were unsure how to report abuse cases. One-half were unsure what state agency was responsible for receiving abuse reports, and over one-third identified the wrong agency. The authors suggest that these and other findings from the study indicate the level of confusion that exists concerning state laws governing elder abuse reporting. Physicians should be more carefully educated about regulations in their state, and mandatory reporting programs should be improved to work better with physicians. Otherwise, efforts to encourage the reporting of suspected abuse will be neutralized.

226   Douglass, Richard L. (1988). *Domestic mistreatment of the elderly: Towards prevention.* Washington, DC: American Association of Retired Persons.

The author explores abuse and neglect of elderly people in home care settings. Five categories of abuse are explained and illustrated with case histories: passive neglect, psychological abuse, material or financial abuse, active neglect, and physical abuse. Intervention in abuse situations usually involves primary prevention, that which takes place at the initial discovery of abuse; and secondary prevention, that which follows initial discovery to prevent further abuse. The author details what individuals, families, and communities can do to prevent elder abuse and neglect with "do" an "don't" lists. The book concludes with a list of available services, and a glossary of related terms.

227   Douglass, Richard L. (July, 1983). Domestic neglect and abuse of the elderly: Implications for research and service. *Family Relations*, 32(3), 395-402.

This article is a review of studies on elder abuse and neglect, and the implications of this research on further study and prevention efforts. Categories of elder abuse have been identified as passive neglect, active neglect, verbal or emotional abuse, and physical abuse. Prevention of abuse and neglect involves increasing the availability of support services for family caregivers, providing meal preparation and housekeeping services, having adequate transportation, giving tax incentives to family caregivers, and other related support systems. The author recommends that future studies are needed to validate already existing data on elder abuse and neglect, and suggests that recognition of elder abuse and appropriate research may allow society to keep this problem from growing.

228   Doyle, Kathleen, & Morrow, Marilyn J. (October-November, 1985). Elder Abuse Awareness Project. *Health Education, 16*(5), 11-13.

      The Illinois Elder Abuse Awareness Project was a study to determine the incidence of elder abuse in several Illinois counties, and to develop, produce, and distribute educational materials to caregivers and senior citizens. A sample of 34 caregivers was given a questionnaire to determine their familiarity with elder abuse and neglect. The most often cited types of neglect were refusal to change bedding or clothes, and refusal to provide proper meals. Other abuses included financial mismanagement and overmedication. Some subjects expressed concern that alcoholism might be a factor in cases of abuse. The subjects also suggested that repeated contact and an emphasis on confidentiality could build trust, and subsequently improve communication. The abused are often reluctant to report abuse, afraid of being put in nursing homes, afraid of change and the unknown, and afraid of being financially dependent. The authors suggest that increased awareness, accurate recognition, and effective intervention in cases of elder abuse should be an integral part of health care workers' and educators' efforts to maintain quality of life and health among the elderly.

229   Fader, Andrew, Koge, Nancy, Gupta, Kilshan L., & Gambert, Steven R. (1990). Perceptions of elder abuse by health care workers in a long-term care setting. *Clinical Gerontologist, 10*(2), 87-89.

      This article is a brief report of a study to examine the attitudes and awareness of long-term care workers toward both passive and active forms of elder abuse. A 17-item questionnaire was completed by 72 randomly selected nursing home workers, including nurse aides, dietitians, physician assistants, physicians, nurses, and allied health workers. Nurse aides scored significantly lower on the test than other groups. Of the nurse aides, those who had worked in long-term care less than five years had lower scores than those who worked in long-term care five years or more.

Nurse aides ages 40 and under also had lower scores, regardless of their years in long-term care. Questions related to passive elder abuse were more frequently missed by all groups completing the test. The authors recommend raising nursing home staff's understanding of elder abuse through ongoing educational efforts.

230   Foelker, George A., Holland, Joan, Marsh, Mary & Simmons, Bobbie A. (1990). A community response to elder abuse. *The Gerontologist, 30*(4), 560-562.

The authors describe the efforts of the Dallas, Texas Area Agency on Aging to meet the 1987 amendments to the Older Americans Act. The amendments required the states to add elder abuse prevention services, and to identify non-profit groups involved in prevention, intervention, and treatment of abuse. A study of elder abuse reports in Dallas revealed that out of 617 reports during 1986 to 1987, 75% were validated, and 48% of these validated cases were successfully resolved. The Elder Abuse Task Force made several conclusions based on the study: 1. the general public and social services were not sufficiently aware of Texas laws concerning elder abuse reporting; 2. the number of reported cases was most likely a small percentage of actual cases of abuse; 3. problems in services to the elderly were due to gaps in services, rather than non-existence of services; 4. the current system was capable of providing intervention services to the abused; 5. neglect by caregivers was a significant factor in the morbidity of clients; 6. the reluctance of victims was a major barrier to abuse intervention; and 7. lack of funding had an adverse effect on the quality and effectiveness of intervention. Based on these conclusions, the state law on elder abuse reporting was amended, and state elder abuse prevention and intervention agencies received more funding.

231   Fulmer, Terry, McMahon, Donald J., Baer-Hines, Maryann, & Forget, Bernadette. (December 1, 1992). Abuse, neglect, abandonment, violence, and exploitation: An analysis of all elderly patients seen in one emergency department during a six-month period. *Journal of Emergency Nursing, 18*(6), 505-510.

The authors studied the charts of all elderly patients (ages 65 and over) admitted to a Connecticut hospital during a six month period to detect evidence of elder abuse and neglect. During the study period, there were 3,153 elderly admissions to the hospital emergency department. There were 1,975 elderly patients admitted during this period, indicating that 63% of the admissions were repeat visits. Neglect was the most prevalent form of abuse (n=70;

3.4%), followed by physical or mental abuse (n=43; 2.3%), violent crime (n=8; 0.4%), abandonment (n=4; 0.2%), and exploitation (n=1, 0.05%). Patient factors significantly associated with abuse were non-white ethnic background, unmarried status, lack of insurance, and documented delirium or dementia.

232   Gallagher, Dolores, Rose, Jonathon, Rivera, Patricia, Lovett, Steven, & Thompson, Larry W. (1989). **Prevalence of depression in family caregivers.** *The Gerontologist, 29*(4), 449-456.

The authors assessed depression in two groups of caregivers: help-seekers (family members who sought help to improve their caregiving skills) and non-help-seekers (family members who volunteered to participate in a study on Alzheimer's disease). The subjects were interviewed using the Schedule for Affective Disorders and Schizophrenia, and all completed the Beck Depression Inventory. Among help-seeking subjects, 46% (31% of men, and 49% of women) met Research Diagnostic Criteria for depression. Among non-help-seeking subjects, 18% met criteria for some type of depressive disorder, with 10% meeting criteria for a major depressive episode. The authors suggest that this type of screening for caregiver depression may effectively identify those caregivers at risk for depression, and that future research is needed to clearly identify the factors which precipitate depression in those who care for the elderly.

233   Giordano, Nan Hervig, & Giordano, Jeffrey A. (May-June, 1984). **Elder abuse: A review of the literature.** *Social Work, 29*(3), 232-236.

The authors review the literature on elder abuse and examine the categories of abuse, the incidence of abuse, and the characteristics of the typical abuse victim. The types of abuse described include physical abuse, negligence, financial exploitation, psychological abuse, violation of rights, and self neglect. Efforts to determine the incidence of abuse have been limited to reports from social service agencies, which are largely inaccurate due to limited reporting laws and a large number of unreported cases. The seven major theoretical explanations of elder abuse are a history of family violence, exposure due to impairment or dependence on caregivers, the personality traits of the abuser, failure to resolve child-parent conflicts, caregiver stress, external stress, and ageism. The typical abuse victim is a severely impaired elderly white woman who is widowed and living with relatives. The authors suggest that future research should use larger samples and focus on the nature, extent, and causes of elder abuse.

234   Godkin, Michael A., Wolf, Rosalie S., & Pillemer, Karl A. (1989). A case-comparison analysis of elder abuse and neglect. *International Journal of Aging and Human Development, 28*(3), 207-225.

This case-control study examined factors which contributed to elderly abuse and neglect by caregivers in a domestic setting. In 59 cases of elder abuse, 40.7% of caregivers had a history of mental health problems, 45.8% had experienced a recent decline in their mental health status, and 20.0% reported a history of problems with alcohol abuse. Based on these and other results, the authors make several conclusions: in cases of abuse and neglect, both caregiver and patient tend to have psychological and emotional problems; the functionally and cognitively impaired elderly are more abused more often; problems in the caregiver-patient relationship play a part in abuse; the lives of the abused are often interrelated to their abusers, often in a shared living environment; and abused elderly are more isolated than non-abused elderly. The combination of emotional problems, dependence, and isolation can create a "pressure-cooker" situation that may lead to abuse. The authors recommend that future research should examine the family dynamics of elder abuse and neglect.

235   Gold, Deborah T., & Gwyther, Lisa P. (January, 1989). The prevention of elder abuse: An educational model. *Family Relations, 38*(1), 8-14.

The authors describe an elder abuse education and prevention curriculum that can be used in community settings, such as senior center programs, Sunday schools, or Rotary meetings. The program includes a discussion of the factors that influence stress and conflict, examples of generational conflicts, a discussion of the appropriate methods for handing conflicts, and information about available support services. The curriculum was pilot tested in North Carolina, Illinois, and Washington, D. C. The authors suggest that this program is an effective way to educate varied groups of people about elder abuse prevention.

236   Griffin, Linner Ward, & Williams, Oliver J. (March, 1992). Abuse among African American elderly. *Journal of Family Violence, 7*(1), 19-36.

The authors describe elder abuse among African Americans. Because research is scarce, and because African American abuse victims do not fit the typical victim profiles promoted by other studies, traditional abuse prevention and intervention programs may be inadequate for this population. The authors suggest that formal and informal groups in the African American community should be educated about the existence and prevention of elder abuse, and that new prevention and intervention programs should use available information about African American patterns of community life, help-seeking, and elder abuse.

237 Hall, Philip A. (1989). Elder maltreatment items, subgroups, and types: Policy and practice implications. *International Journal of Aging and Human Development, 28*(3), 191-205.

The author studied 284 validated cases of elder abuse to discover what factors were used to validate reported abuse. Validation of reported abuse involves discovering whether Department of Human Rights criteria exist in the situation. The elements that occurred most often in the study cases were neglect of patient environment and/or medical care. Exploitation of financial resources and verbal aggression were also seen in many cases. More than one element of abuse was found in 69.4% of the cases. Based on the findings of the study, the author discusses the implications of current policy and practice in cases of elder abuse.

238 Hickey, Tom, & Douglass, Richard L. (1981). Neglect and abuse of older family members: Professionals' perspectives and case experiences. *The Gerontologist, 21*(2), 171-176.

The authors interviewed 228 health care professionals, police officers, lawyers, caseworkers, clergy, morticians, and coroners about their experiences with elder abuse and neglect. Nearly all of the subjects had firsthand experience with passive neglect, but only a few of them considered it a critical problem. Only 77 of the subjects reported having no experience with physical abuse, and almost none of the subjects were unfamiliar with any other type of abuse. The professionals' explanations of the causes of neglect and abuse were varied. The authors suggest that a causal model free of professional bias is needed to accurately detect elder abuse.

239 Homer, Ann C., & Gilleard, C. (December 15, 1990). Abuse of elderly people by their carers. *British Medical Journal, 301*(6765), 1359-1362.

This British study collected information on abuse and risk factors for abuse to assess the prevalence of elder abuse and the characteristics of abusers and their victims. Over a period of six months, the authors interviewed 51 caregivers, and found that 45% of caregivers admitted some form of abuse: 27% admitted to one type, 14% to two types, and 3% to all three types of abuse (physical abuse, verbal abuse, and neglect). Results indicated that some of the commonly accepted signs of elder abuse were not necessarily associated with abuse, such as bruising or social isolation. The most significant risk factors for abuse were use of alcohol by the caregiver and problematic long-term relationships. The authors suggest that family care for elderly may not be the best option in at-risk families.

240   Huston, Patricia G. (September, 1990). Family care of the elderly and caregiver stress. *American Family Physician, 42*(3), 671-676.

The author describes the family caregiver, usually a child or a spouse, and explains the stress involved in caring for a family member. Caregiver stress, if extreme and untreated, may lead to elder abuse. Primary physicians can help caregivers deal with stress by providing emotional support, educating caregivers about support services, giving advice, and intervening in cases of suspected abuse. The author suggests that supportive family physicians can help reduce caregiver stress and prevent subsequent elder abuse.

241   Jorgensen, Jay E. (March-April, 1993). An intervention program for dentists to detect elder abuse and neglect. *Public Health Reports, 108*(2), 171-172.

This article describes an intervention program to determine dentists' awareness of and attitudes toward reporting elder abuse. Three groups of dentists in California will participate in the program: a control group, an intervention group, and an intervention and self-monitoring group. The groups will complete a questionnaire to determine their awareness of and ability to detect elder abuse and their willingness to report possible cases of abuse. The intervention will be a two-hour presentation of signs and symptoms of elder abuse. After six months, all three groups will be surveyed about any abuse cases detected in their practice.

242   Kosberg, Jordan I. (Ed.). (1983). *Abuse and maltreatment of the elderly: Causes and interventions.* Boston: John Wright • PSG Inc.

This book is a collection of articles by experts in the field of elder abuse and neglect. Topics include victimology, the fear of crime, personal crimes against the elderly, the consequences of institutionalization, fraud and abuse in nursing homes, domestic neglect and abuse, dependence, stress, violence between middle-aged caregivers and elderly parents, victimization by health professionals, and federal legislation.

243   Kosberg, Jordan I. (February, 1988). **Preventing elder abuse: Identification of high risk factors prior to placement decisions.** *The Gerontologist, 28*(1), 43-50.

The author discusses prevention of elder abuse, especially in relation to placement decisions. Elder abuse may go unreported because professionals are reluctant to interfere in family problems, because the abuse may occur in isolated settings, because the elderly are reluctant to report abuse, because professionals are unaware of the problem, and because professionals do not report abuse. Assessment of a proposed caregiving environment for elder abuse risk factors may prevent the placement of an elderly person in a high-risk environment. Factors identifying vulnerable elderly include female gender, advanced age, dependence, problem drinking, intergenerational conflict, internalizing blame, excessive loyalty, a history of abuse, stoicism, isolation, impairment, and provocative behavior. High-risk caregivers are often substance (alcohol, drugs, or prescription medication) abusers, impaired by senile dementia or confusion, mentally or emotionally ill, inexperienced, economically troubled, abused in the past, stressed, isolated at home, prone to blaming others, unsympathetic, lacking understanding, economically dependent, or hypercritical. Risk factors in family environments include lack of family support, reluctance to provide care, overcrowding, isolation, marital problems, economic pressures, family problems, a desire to institutionalize the patient, and a lack of agreement about responsibility for care. The author suggests that identifying the existence of these risk factors in a pre-placement screening can help professionals prevent placing the elderly in situations conducive to abuse.

244   Lachs, Mark S., & Fulmer, Terry. (August, 1993). **Recognizing elder abuse and neglect.** *Clinics in Geriatric Medicine, 9*(3), 665-682.

The authors discuss elder abuse and neglect, emphasizing procedures for assessing and evaluating reports or suspicion of abuse. Screening for elder abuse can be difficult, because the symptoms may be hidden or consistent with other, more common medical conditions. Performing a complete assessment involves taking separate medical histories from patient and caregiver, as well as performing clinical assessments of physical, cognitive, and functional abilities. If abuse is detected, management, reporting, and intervention pose difficult ethical and legal problems. The authors recommend that clinicians remove patients from immediate danger situations. In less acute cases, appropriate intervention to remove risk factors is appropriate. The article includes a sample assessment protocol as an appendix.

245   Marson, Stephen M. (1993). The Mental Status Questionnaire in cases of elder neglect and abuse. *Clinical Gerontologist, 12*(4), 61-64.

This article describes two cases in which the author used the Mental Status Questionnaire to evaluate charges of elder abuse and neglect in a nursing home setting. In both cases, the Mental Status Questionnaire proved useful in determining the patient's level of confusion. Despite the fact that level of confusion could not be used to fully determine the veracity of the charges, the author recommends using the Mental Status Questionnaire in such cases to assess patient credibility.

246   Moon, Ailee, & Williams, Oliver. (June, 1993). Perceptions of elder abuse and help-seeking patterns among African-American, Caucasian American, and Korean-American elderly women. *The Gerontologist, 33*(3), 386-395.

This study examined ethnic differences in perceptions of elder abuse and patterns of help-seeking. Subjects were 30 African American, 30 Korean American, and 30 Caucasian American elderly women (ages 60 and over). The researchers described 13 scenarios and asked each subject if the situations involved abuse. If the subject answered yes, they were asked to list the aspects of the situations that involved abuse, and to rate the severity of the abuse. In all scenarios, subjects were asked if they would have asked for help if they were the elderly person in the scenario. If the answer was yes, they were asked to identify who they would have asked for help. The Korean American subjects were more likely than the other groups to have a narrow definition of abuse, and to express both their reluctance to cause "family shame" and their fear of causing family conflict by reporting abuse. Because the sample was small, and limited to women, the authors caution against over-generalizing the results of the study, but suggest that future research should investigate the elderly person's ability to perceive situations of abuse, and the ethnic or cultural influences on perceptions of abuse and help-seeking.

247 Ogg, Jim, & Munn-Giddings, Carol. (September, 1993). Researching elder abuse. *Ageing and Society, 13*(3), 389-414.

This article compares American research on elder abuse with similar research in Britain and Canada. Previous studies have been limited by methodology relying on self-reports and mandatory reporting programs. While most of the research has been focused on the characteristics of the abused and the abuser, the authors suggest that future research should also consider the sociological dimensions of elder abuse.

248 Paveza, Gregory J., Cohen, Donna, Eisdorfer, Carl, Freels, Sally, Semla, Todd, Ashford, J. Wesson, Gorelick, Philip, Hirschman, Robert, Luchins, Daniel & Levy, Paul. (August, 1992). Severe family violence and Alzheimer's disease: Prevalence and risk factors. *The Gerontologist, 32*(4), 493-497.

This study assessed the prevalence of violence and the risk factors for violence associated with Alzheimer's disease patients in a community setting. Subjects were 184 Alzheimer's disease patients and their caregivers. The Conflict Tactics Scale was used to identify levels of violence. In the year since diagnosis, 15.8% of the patients had been violent, and 5.4% of the caregivers reported being violent toward their patients. Two variables were significantly associated with violence: caregiver depression and living with family but without a spouse. The authors recommend that current studies should be followed by longitudinal studies to determine whether identified risk factors are correct, and to more accurately determine rates of prevalence and incidence.

249 Pillemer, Karl & Finkelhor, David. (1988). The prevalence of elder abuse: A random sample survey. *The Gerontologist, 28*(1), 51-57.

This large-scale, random sample survey of elder abuse and neglect was designed to assess the prevalence and nature of elder abuse in the community. Subjects were 2,020 community-dwelling elderly in Boston. Interviews were conducted in two stages: an initial screening to detect elder abuse, and a follow-up interview with those deemed abuse victims. The prevalence rate was 32 victims per 1,000 elderly, but only 1 in 14 cases came to public attention. Spouses were found to be the most likely abusers. The numbers of male and female victims were nearly equal, but women suffered more serious abuse. These results indicate that under-reporting of elder abuse is substantial, and that spousal abuse is common in this population. The authors suggest that existing service programs for caregivers and the abused need to be changed to reflect these findings.

250   Pillemer, Karl, & Finkelhor, David. (April, 1989). Causes of elder abuse: Caregiver stress versus problem relatives. *American Journal of Orthopsychiatry, 59*(2), 179-187.

This study examined abused elderly to determine whether elder abuse was caused by caregiver stress or by problem caregivers. A survey of Boston area elderly (ages 65 and over) identified 61 abused elderly. Victims were most often abused by their spouses: 60% of physical abuse and 58% of maltreatment was perpetrated by a spouse. Abusers were more likely to have a history of socioemotional problems than non-abusers, and were more likely dependent on their patients. The factors that tended to identify abusive situations were related to the caregiver's behaviors or circumstances, and not related to the health or dependence of the victim. The characteristics of the caregiver, such as emotional problems or deviant behavior, were better predictors of abuse than the dependence or disability of the patient. Abusers appear to be severely troubled, with histories of anti-social or unstable behavior. The authors conclude that the picture of elder abuse as the result of an overburdened caregiver is, in fact, the opposite of most abusive situations, and recommend that intervention should be directed at the emotional and behavioral problems of the caregivers.

251   Pillemer, Karl, & Hudson, Beth. (February, 1993). A model abuse prevention program for nursing assistants. *The Gerontologist, 33*(1), 128-131.

The authors developed an interactive abuse prevention curriculum for nursing home assistants at 10 Philadelphia nursing homes. The program contains eight modules: 1. a general overview of abuse in nursing homes, 2. an explanation of the different types of abuse, 3. a discussion of what causes abuse, 4. a discussion and evaluation of participants' stress, 5. a review of the impact of culture and ethnicity on conflicts with patients, 6. a discussion of patient aggression, 7. a discussion of ethical issues concerning reporting abuse, and 8. a review of strategies to prevent abuse. The program was well-received at the 10 test sites, and posttest results showed improvements in several indicators, including reduced levels of conflict. The authors suggest that similar programs should be included as basic training for nursing home staff.

252   Pillemer, Karl, & Moore, David W. (1989). **Abuse of patients in nursing homes: Findings from a survey of staff.** *The Gerontologist, 29*(3), 314-320.

This study examined the rates of abuse and risk factors for abuse in intermediate care and skilled nursing facilities. Subjects were 577 staff from 31 nursing facilities. The subjects were interviewed by telephone, and asked to describe what types of abuse they had seen, and what types of abuse they had committed themselves. Findings showed that 36% of subjects had seen at least one situation of physical abuse in the past year. Over-use of restraints was the most common type of physical abuse, reported by 21% of subjects, followed by pushing, grabbing, shoving, or pinching (17%), slapping or hitting (12%), throwing things (3%), kicking or hitting with a fist (2%), and hitting with an object (2%). Psychological abuse was seen by 81% of subjects. Reported psychological abuse included yelling (70%), intentional isolation (23%), threats of violence (15%), and denying food or privileges (13%). When asked which types of behavior they had committed, 10% admitted committing one or more physically abusive acts in the previous year, and 40% reported at least one psychologically abusive act. The survey also indicated that abusers were more likely to have a stressful working environment, negative attitudes toward the elderly, and emotional problems. The authors suggest that reducing stress and training staff to resolve conflicts will improve quality of life for residents of nursing homes.

253   Powell, Sharon, & Berg, Robert C. (1987). **When the elderly are abused: Characteristics and intervention.** *Educational Gerontology, 13*(1), 71-83.

This study examined the characteristics of the elder abuse victims and abusers, the types and duration of abuse, descriptions of abusive situations, the reporting and verification of abuse, case management strategies utilized by caseworkers, and the consequences of those strategies. Subjects were 60 elder abuse cases selected from the files of an Adult Protective Services unit. The study showed that victims were more likely ages 75 and over and female. A majority of the victims (80%) lived in their own homes. Passive neglect was seen in only 3% of the cases, which may indicate that passive forms of abuse are harder to detect, and seldom reported. Financial abuse was the most common (61.7%), followed by emotional abuse (55%), physical abuse (45%), and active neglect (35%). Only 2 out of the 60 cases of abuse were reported as isolated incidents. Reports of abuse were most often made by someone other than the victim (81.7%), usually relatives, friends, or neighbors (31.7%). In at least 48% of cases, relatives were aware of the abuse, but less than 17% of reports came from relatives. Caseworker strategies were varied, but usually included legal services such as restraining orders, mental health warrants, or reports to law enforcement. The authors conclude that elder abuse is an often unreported, complex, and widespread problem, and recommend that further research improve screening for abuse, and routes for access and intervention in situations of abuse.

254   Pritchard, Jacki. (1992). *The abuse of elderly people: A handbook for professionals.* Philadelphia: Jessica Kingsley Publishers.

This book includes the following topics: definitions of abuse, how to recognize abuse, working with abuse, basic facts about abuse, and what it's like to be abused. Pritchard defines abuse as any misuse, perversion, unjust or corrupt practice, reviling, insulting or unkind speech. Guidelines for recognizing and preventing abuse are suggested in four areas: physical abuse, psychological abuse, sociological abuse, and legal abuse.

255   Quinn, Mary Joy, & Tomita, Susan K. (1986). *Elder abuse and neglect.* New York: Springer Publishing Company.

The authors describe the phenomenon of elder abuse and neglect, elder abuse diagnosis and intervention, practice issues, and future directions. According to the authors, the typical victim of elder abuse and neglect is a woman. The text includes numerous case examples.

256   Scharlach, Andrew E. (June, 1989). A comparison of employed caregivers of cognitively impaired and physically impaired elderly persons. *Research on Aging, 11*(2), 225-243.

This study examined the consequences of combining work and caregiving in 332 employees of a California insurance company. The subjects reported that they were caregivers to an elderly person (ages 60 and over). Subjects who cared for cognitively impaired patients were more likely to report higher levels of stress, and negative effects on their personal and social activities. They were also more likely to seek nursing home placement within the next two years. Employees who were caregivers to the cognitively impaired were more likely to have a conflict between their work and caregiving. Programs considered helpful were those providing information about available community services, support groups, and personal counseling. The authors suggest that future research should examine the relationship between work and caregiver stress, especially for caregivers of cognitively impaired patients.

257 Schlesinger, Benjamin, & Schlesinger, Rachel, (Eds.). (1988). *Abuse of the elderly: Issues and annotated bibliography.* Toronto: University of Toronto Press.

This book includes articles by several writers on the following topics: grannybashing, the impact of abuse on hospital social work, assessment, and the protection of elderly mentally incompetent individuals who are often victims of abuse.

258 Shiferaw, Beletshachew, Mittlemark, Maurice B., Wofford, James L., Anderson, Roger T., Walls, Princilla, & Rohrer, Brenda. (February, 1994). The investigation and outcome of reported cases of elder abuse: The Forsyth County aging study. *The Gerontologist, 34*(1), 123-125.

This study examined elder abuse investigations in Forsyth County, North Carolina. During a three-year period, there were 123 investigations, 23 of which were confirmed as elder abuse. There were no statistically significant differences between the gender, age, and other factors of confirmed versus nonconfirmed reports of abuse. The low percentage of confirmed cases may be due to failure of the investigation, investigators' different definitions of abuse, and false reports. The authors suggest that future studies should use standard definitions of abuse and thoroughly investigate reported cases for both false positives and false-negatives.

259 Skipwith, Delois Hughes. (March, 1994). Telephone counseling interventions with caregivers of elders. *Journal of Psychosocial Nursing and Mental Health Services, 32*(3), 7-12.

This article describes a program to help caregivers cope with the stress of caregiving through brief interventions over the telephone. The counseling was designed to help caregivers cope with caregiving, gain confidence in problem-solving, find and use support services, and solve conflicts appropriately. The sessions lasted 15 minutes, and calls were made three times per week. The author describes four cases, giving details of the subjects' reported caregiving problems, and the interventions suggested in each situation. Interventions were usually exploring other options for care, maintaining the support of family members, providing information, supporting religious beliefs, exploring other sources of help, solving problems, and supporting the caregiver. The author suggests that telephone counseling may be an economical and efficient method of intervention to reduce caregiver stress.

260   Stiegel, Lori A., Norrgard, Lee, & Talbert, Robin. (October, 1992). Scams in the marketing and sale of living trusts: A new fraud for the 1990s. *Clearinghouse Review, 26*(6), 609-612.

The authors discuss living trusts, which are complicated legal documents used in estate planning. Companies marketing these trusts have reportedly made false claims about the tax and cost savings of these plans, their ability as nonlawyers to correctly and legally complete the documents, as well as their connections to reputable organizations. The documents are often incomplete or ineffective because of error. The elderly are particularly at risk for this kind of fraud, because they are more interested in, yet less knowledgeable about, issues of probate and guardianship of their finances. They may also be reluctant or unable to hire an attorney. Several state attorney generals have investigated these companies, and have pursued civil and criminal lawsuits. At least two state supreme courts have prohibited the sale of living trusts by nonlawyers as an unauthorized practice of law.

261   Strumpf, Neville E., & Evans, Lois K. (1991). The ethical problems of prolonged physical restraint. *Journal of Gerontological Nursing, 17*(2).

This article describes the many ethical problems associated with using physical restraints in nursing homes and care facilities. These restraints may include anything from vests and mitts to wrist ties and locked chairs. The authors describe three cases of restraint use to illustrate a difficult subject, and dispute several myths supporting the use of restraints. The authors suggest that restraints should rarely be used, if ever. Instead, appropriate patient management and injury prevention should include simpler methods that are available, effective, and have a smaller impact on quality of life for elderly patients.

262 Weiner, Adele. (Fall-Winter, 1991). A community-based education model for identification and prevention of elder abuse. *Journal of Gerontological Social Work, 16*(3-4), 107-120.

This article describes the Brooklyn Elder Abuse Training Project, which targeted professionals, community leaders, the elderly, and families. The project used a series of workshops and consultations to make the targeted groups aware of elder abuse, and to discuss the issues related to identification and reporting of abuse. Because the program clarified the roles of each of the targeted groups in abuse intervention, the program will facilitate the process of identifying, reporting, and dealing with cases of abuse. The author suggests that formal programs of elder abuse education will improve the delivery of services to the elderly, especially those in otherwise unreported situations of abuse.

263 Weith, Mel E. (February, 1994). Elder abuse: A national tragedy. *FBI Law Enforcement Bulletin, 63*(2), 24-27.

The author discusses the responsibility of law enforcement in cases of elder abuse. Because the number of recognized cases of abuse is growing, and many cases are still going unreported, new and veteran law enforcement officers must be trained in basic gerontology and the warning signs of abuse. The most successful method of elder abuse prevention is eliminating the probability of mistreatment. The author suggests that law enforcement officers, if properly trained, can adequately identify and intervene in cases of abuse for this at-risk population.

264 Wolf, Rosalie S., & Pillemer, Karl. (February, 1994). What's new in elder abuse programming? Four bright ideas. *The Gerontologist, 34*(1), 126-129.

The authors describe four community elder abuse programs. In California, a multidisciplinary team of professionals meets monthly to review and assess elder abuse cases. Established protocols include suggested interventions, follow-up on the team's recommendations in each case, and follow-up on action taken in each case. In Wisconsin, a group of volunteer advocates provide a link to support services, advocacy, and emotional support in cases of abuse. The volunteers are trained by the local Area Agency on Aging and cooperated with both elder abuse specialists and domestic violence programs. A victim support group in New York is used to create a network of support for abuse victims, who meet on a regular basis. This "buddy system" allows the members to remain connected to a group and to avoid the isolation often associated with abusive situations. In Hawaii, the state university offered a master's level social work program in conjunction with Adult Protective Services. The students were trained and used as a unit to participate in the investigation and evaluation of reported cases of abuse. The authors suggest that these programs were successful because they were appropriate for the urban areas they served, and because they were supported by local adult protective and human services.

7

Falls

Falls are the second leading cause of accidental death among elderly people ages 55 to 79. For people ages 80 and over, falls become the leading cause of death. In addition to fatalities, falls are responsible for many other injuries which threaten the independence of older people and cause a substantial proportion of all hospitalizations of older adults. This chapter includes articles and books providing information about prevalence, risk factors, hazards, and prevention interventions. Settings for empirical research include the community, residential care facilities, and nursing homes. Articles are also included which deal with consequences of falls, such as hip fractures and head injuries.

265 Acton, Patricia A., Farley, Thomas, Freni, Lambertina W., Ilegbodu, Victor A., Sniezek, Joseph E., & Wohlleb, James C. (October, 1993). Traumatic spinal cord injury in Arkansas, 1980 to 1989. *Archives of Physical Medicine and Rehabilitation, 74*(10), 1035-1040.

Using data from the Arkansas State Spinal Cord Commission (ASSCC) registry, the authors studied the causes of and groups of people affected by spinal cord injuries (SCI) in Arkansas since 1977. Overall, transportation-related incidents were responsible for 49.5% of SCI. Males ages 15 to 24 were most likely to suffer SCI due to a higher prevalence of sports- and transportation-related injuries. Minority males ages 15 to 44 were at the highest risk for violence-related SCI. Among elderly people (ages 65 and over), the rate of SCI from falls was 2.8 times higher than for younger people. The authors recommend further intervention to prevent injuries in these groups.

266   Alexander, Bruce H., Rivara, Frederick P., & Wolf, Marsha E. (July, 1992). **The cost and frequency of hospitalization for fall-related injuries in older adults.** *American Journal of Public Health, 82*(7), 1020-1023.

This study examined hospitalizations of older adults in Washington State during 1989 for fall-related injuries. Fall-related injuries made up 5.3% of all hospitalizations of older adults, with hospital charges totaling $53,346,191. These hospitalizations also resulted in discharge to nursing care more often than other types of injuries. The annual hospitalization rate was 13.5 per 1,000 persons, with an annual cost of $92 per person. The authors recommend further study to develop low-cost, brief interventions that could effectively decrease both the risk and frequency of falls in this population.

267   Arfken, Cynthia L., Lach, Helen W., Birge, Stanley J., & Miller, J. Philip. (April, 1994). **The prevalence and correlates of fear of falling in elderly persons living in the community.** *American Journal of Public Health, 84*(4), 565-570.

This article describes a study to assess prevalence of fear of falling and its association with falling, quality of life, and frailty in elderly people. Prevalence and association were determined from a follow-up study of subjects (gender- and age-stratified random sample of 1,358 community-dwelling elderly) from a parent study on physician screening for falls. The authors found that fear of falling was common among this sample. Prevalence increased with age, and was higher in women. Factors associated with fear of falling (after adjustment for age and gender) were decreased life satisfaction, increased frailty, depressed mood, and recent experience with falls.

268   Brody, Elaine M., Kleban, Morton H., Moss, Miriam S., & Kleban, Ferne. (1984). **Predictors of falls among institutionalized women with Alzheimer's disease.** *Journal of the American Geriatrics Society, 32*(12), 877-882.

This study analyzed a group of 60 institutionalized women with senile dementia of the Alzheimer type (mean age 83 years) to determine whether low levels of physical vigor and declines in vigor were associated with the occurrence and frequency of falls. Subjects were studied longitudinally and evaluated annually on 21 variables of physical, social, emotional, self-care, and cognitive functioning. A substudy of the subjects' subsequent falls used data from two of these evaluations. Clinical ratings by the researchers estimated changes in function during the preceding year and current levels of functioning. Separate regressions for each of the two years returned identical significant patterns, indicating that physical vigor was significantly related to number of falls. The women who had been among the most vigorous in the group, but who had shown significant declines in the preceding year, were the most vulnerable to falls. Those who had been rated as the least vigorous, but whose levels of vigor had been stable during the year, tended to have fewer falls. These results show that falling appears to be related to the process of decline in vigor among those whose levels of vigor were initially higher. There were also corresponding declines in emotional and cognitive scales.

269   Buchner, David M., & Larson, Eric B. (March 20, 1987). **Falls and fractures in patients with Alzheimer-type dementia.** *Journal of the American Medical Association, 257*(11), 1492-1495.

This study analyzed the morbidity, mortality, and risks for falls in elderly patients with Alzheimer-type dementia (ATD). Subjects were 157 ATD patients ages 62 and over (mean age 79 years). At the initial evaluation, 4% lived in nursing homes, 31% reported falls, and only one subject was unable to walk. During the three-year follow-up period, 59% of the 117 follow-up subjects were placed in nursing homes, and over 50% either fell or became unable to walk. Overall mortality was 26%. The rate of fracture during follow-up was more than three times the age- and gender-adjusted fracture rate for the general population. Risk factors associated with ATD were impaired gait, impaired balance, and wandering. Other risks were associated with comorbid illness: poor vision, arthritis, and toxic drug reactions. The authors recommend that strategies to prevent toxic drug reactions, to treat comorbid illness, to control wandering, and to manage the environments of ATD patients may all help reduce the risk of falls in this population.

270   Campbell, A. John, Borrie, Michael J., & Spears, George F. (1989). **Risk factors for falls in a community-based prospective study of people 70 years and older.** *Journals of Gerontology, 44*(4), M112-M117.

This study investigated factors associated with falls in a New Zealand community-based prospective study of 761 elderly subjects (ages 70 and over). The subjects were assessed to identify various physical and demographic variables. The group experienced 507 falls during the following year of study. Variables associated with an increased risk of falling differed in men and women. For men, decreased levels of physical activity, stroke, arthritis of the knees, impairment of gait, and increased body sway were associated with an increased risk of falls. In women, the total number of drugs, psychotropic drugs, drugs liable to cause postural hypotension, low standing systolic blood pressure, and evidence of muscle weakness were also associated with an increased risk of falling. The authors conclude that most falls in elderly people are associated with multiple risk factors, many of which are potentially remediable, and suggest an approach to prevention. After taking a full history of a fall, the clinician should determine whether the cause was internal or external. If external, then advice should be given about potentially hazardous activities. If internal, the clinician should isolate the often multiple factors and correct as many as possible.

271   Catchen, Hervey. (September, 1987). Consequence of patient accident reports for the frail elderly. *Journal of Applied Gerontology, 6*(3), 284-299.

This study looks at procedures for preparing accident reports in a nursing facility. Catchen analyzed the content of 392 accident reports and interviews with 51 elderly accident victims. The author reports that wheelchairs and beds were associated with over half of all accidents. The data analysis indicated that a small group of people (mostly males) had experienced multiple accidents. From the samples presented in the article, many falls appear to be associated with people getting out of bed or out of chairs to go to the bathroom. The author concluded that many incidents reported as accidents in hospitals would pass as minor, insignificant events. In a large majority of the reports reviewed by Catchen, the patients did not experience an injury as a result of the accident.

272   Chapuy, Marie C., Arlot, Monique E., Duboeuf, Francois, Brun, Jacqueline, Crouzet, Brigitte, Arnaud, Simone, Delmas, Pierre D., & Meunier, Pierre J. (December 3, 1992). Vitamin D3 and calcium to prevent hip fractures in elderly women. *New England Journal of Medicine, 327*(23), 1637-1642.

This study examined the effects of supplementation with vitamin D3 (cholecalciferol) and calcium on the frequency of hip fractures and other nonvertebral fractures. Subjects were 3,270 healthy, ambulatory women (mean age 84 years). Each day for 18 months, 1,634 women received tricalcium phosphate and vitamin D3, and 1,636 women received a double placebo. Among the women who completed the 18-month study, the number of hip fractures was 43% lower (p = .043) and the total number of nonvertebral fractures was 32% lower (p = .015) among the women treated with vitamin D3 and calcium than among those who received the placebo. The bone density of the proximal femur increased 2.7% in the vitamin D3/calcium group and decreased 4.6% in the placebo group (p < .001). The authors conclude that vitamin D3 and calcium supplements reduce the risk of hip fractures and other nonvertebral fractures among elderly women.

273   Chen, Hsieh-Ching, Ashton-Miller, James A., Alexander, Neil B., & Schultz, Albert B. (November, 1991). Stepping over obstacles: Gait patterns of healthy young and old adults. *Journals of Gerontology, 46*(6), M196-M203.

This article describes a study that analyzed gait patterns of healthy young men and women and healthy old men and women as they approached and stepped over obstacles of various heights. Subjects were 48 volunteers (12 young males, 12 young females, 12 old males, 12 old females) who were monitored electronically as they walked along a path with obstacles ranging in height from standard door thresholds up to the average curbstone. Each of the volunteers walked the course 42 times. The old adults were more conservative when crossing obstacles than young adults. All subjects avoided tripping on or kicking the obstacle. Four of the old adults stepped on the obstacle. Attention and cognition were not measured in this study, and the artificial setting may not reflect what happens when people walk in everyday settings. The results of the study indicate that old adults are more careful when stepping over obstacles than young adults.

274   Cinque, Chris. (August, 1990). Women's strength training: Lifting the limits of aging? *The Physician and Sportsmedicine, 18*(8), 123-127.

This article reviews weight training that doctors are now prescribing to alleviate back and muscle problems in women. The benefits of strength training include more than just physical conditioning. Training can also reduce injury, increase confidence, and preserve some of the flexibility that often deteriorates with age. Weight training can even benefit women who already have osteoporosis by helping them develop their overall strength and muscle tone.

275 Clark, Russell D., Lord, Stephen R., & Webster, Ian W. (March, 1993). **Clinical parameters associated with falls in an elderly population.** *Gerontology, 39*(2), 117-123.

This study was conducted at an Australian hostel for the aged to determine whether clinical examinations of elderly people could predict risk factors for falls. The 81 subjects, ages 70 to 97 (mean age 83.3 years), were examined with an emphasis on measures of posture, balance, and gait. The subjects' muscular, visual, cardiovascular, and neurological function were also examined, and a history of medical conditions and medication use was taken. To assess which of these clinical measures were associated with future falls, 76 subjects were followed-up for one year, of which 34 (44.7%) reported no falls. Of those who fell, 10 (13.2%) fell once, 13 (17.1%) fell twice, and 19 (25.0%) fell three or more times. The majority (72.0%) of falls occurred inside the hostel building, which had already been modified to minimize environmental hazards. Stepwise logistic regression analysis was used to evaluate which clinical factors could most correctly identify fallers. Four major factors were identified: impaired cognition, abnormal reaction to any push or pressure, history of palpitations, and abnormal stepping. The authors conclude that clinical examination focused on these areas could be useful for assessment of risk and prediction of falls.

276 Cooper, C., Barker, D. J. P., & Wickham, C. (December 3, 1988). **Physical activity, muscle strength, and calcium intake in fracture of the proximal femur in Britain.** *British Medical Journal, 297*(6661), 1443-1446.

The authors studied the role of regular exercise and high calcium intake in preventing hip fracture. The physical activity and calcium intake of 300 British elderly men and women (ages 50 and over) with hip fractures were compared with those of 600 controls matched for age and gender. For both men and women, increased daily activity, including standing, walking, climbing stairs, carrying, housework, and gardening protected against fracture. This effect was independent of other known risk factors, including body mass, cigarette smoking, and alcohol consumption. Strength of grip correlated with activity and was inversely related to the risk of fracture. Calcium intake was not related to the risk of fracture in women. Men with daily calcium intakes above 1 gram had lower risks. The authors suggest that these findings point to the importance of elderly people in Britain maintaining physical activity in their day-to-day lives.

277 Cumming, Robert G., & Klineberg, Robin J. (March 1, 1994). Case-control study of risk factors for hip fractures in the elderly. *American Journal of Epidemiology, 139*(5), 493-503.

This study investigated risk factors for hip fractures in the elderly with an emphasis on factors occurring during young and middle adult life. The 416 (209 cases, 207 controls) subjects ages 65 and over were recruited from hospitals and nursing homes, and from the general community in Sydney, Australia. Factors associated with increased risk of hip fracture included low relative weight in old age, physical inactivity in old age, history of smoking, and psychotropic medications. The study also showed that consumption of dairy products at age 20 may also increase the risk for hip fracture, a finding which the authors think may be due to chance or bias in the sample. If confirmed by further study, this finding may challenge current injury prevention efforts. The study is consistent, however, with previous studies that suggest reduction of hip fracture risk may be attained by being physically active, maintaining healthy weight, and stopping smoking.

278 Cumming, Robert G., Miller, J. Philip, Kelsey, Jennifer L., Davis, Paula, Arfken, Cynthia L., Birge, Stanley J., & Peck, William. (November, 1991). Medications and multiple falls in elderly people: The St. Louis OASIS Study. *Age and Ageing, 20*(6), 455-461.

The authors studied the relationship between commonly prescribed medications and the risk of falls in an elderly population. Subjects were 1,358 functionally independent, community-dwelling elderly (ages 65 and over) from an educational organization in St. Louis, Missouri. Subjects reported their history of falls in the past year, as well as their use of medications. Findings showed that 27% of subjects reported at least one fall in the past year, and 8% reported two or more falls. Medications shown to increase risk for multiple falls included diazepam, diltiazem, diuretics, and laxatives. The authors recommend that physicians prescribe these medications to elderly patients with great caution.

279   Cummings, Steven R., & Nevitt, Michael C. (1989). A hypothesis: The cause of hip fractures. *Journals of Gerontology, 44*(4), M107-M111.

This article describes the authors' theory of those factors which influence the increase of hip fracture with age. They propose that four conditions must be satisfied in order for a fall to cause a hip fracture: 1. the faller must be oriented to impact near the hip; 2. protective responses must fail; 3. local soft tissues must absorb less energy than necessary to prevent fracture; and 4. the residual energy of the fall applied to the proximal femur must exceed its strength. These events become more likely with age and lead to the exponential rise in the risk of hip fracture with advancing age. This model may also suggest that a combination of measurements of neuromuscular function and of bone strength may be the most accurate way to assess the risk of hip fracture.

280   Cummings, Steven R., Nevitt, Michael C., & Kidd, Sharon. (July, 1988). Forgetting falls: The limited accuracy of recall of fall in the elderly. *Journal of the American Geriatrics Society, 36*(7), 613-616.

This study examined the accuracy of elderly subjects' recollections of recent falls. Subjects were 304 ambulatory elderly men and women (ages 60 and over) who completed a 12-month prospective study of risk factors for falling. A system of weekly follow-up and home visits recorded and confirmed all falls. During the study, 179 subjects suffered at least one confirmed fall. At the end of the study, all subjects were asked by telephone if they had fallen during the previous 3, 6, or 12 months. Depending on the time period of recall, 13% to 32% of those with confirmed falls did not recall falling during the specific period of time. Recall was better for the preceding 12 months than for 3 or 6 months. There were only weak correlations between the documented and recalled falls. Those with lower scores on the Mini–Mental State Examination were more likely to forget falls. The authors conclude that the elderly often do not recall falls that occurred during specific periods of time over the preceding 3 to 12 months, and recommend that researchers and clinicians consider using methods other than long-term recall to ascertain and count falls over specific periods of time.

281   Davie, James W., Blumenthal, Monica D., & Robinson-Hawkins, Susan. (April, 1981). A model of risk of falling for psychogeriatric patients. *Archives of General Psychiatry, 38*, 463-467.

This study examined 100 community-dwelling psychiatric outpatients, ages 60 and over, for factors associated with symptoms of dizziness, falling, and orthostatic hypotension. Of the subjects, 39% complained of dizziness or falling, and 34% had systolic orthostatic hypotension. The combination of systolic and diastolic blood pressure drop, type of somatic illness, type and number of drugs, and psychiatric diagnosis accounted for 50% of the variance in dizziness and falling. Type of illness, drug category, and psychiatric diagnosis accounted for only 19% of the variance in orthostatic hypotension. Statistical analysis showed that systolic orthostatic hypotension, disease classification, and type and number of drugs taken all contributed independently to dizziness and falling. The authors recommend that, in geriatric psychiatric patients, careful attention to orthostatic hypotension, concurrent somatic illness, and number and type of medications is essential to the prevention of dizziness and falling.

282 DeVito, Carolee A., Lambert, Deborah A., Sattin, Richard W., Bacchelli, Sandro, Ros, Alberto, & Rodriguez, Juan G. (November, 1988). Fall injuries among the elderly: Community-based surveillance. *Journal of the American Geriatrics Society*, 36(11), 1029-1035.

The authors established a community-based surveillance system in Miami Beach, Florida, as part of a study to assess falls among the elderly. A total of 1,827 fall injury events occurred in this community between July, 1985 and June, 1986. Over 85% (1,567) of the fall injuries were identified by emergency room records. The remaining cases were identified from fire rescue reports, inpatient medical records, or medical examiner reports. Accidental falls were most common (97%). More than 100 people sought medical assistance from a fall each month. Time of injury was known for 68% of those who fell. A majority of these falls (94%) occurred during daylight hours. Over half of the falls (54%) occurred in and around the home, and 38% of these had a particular area of the home recorded: 42% occurred in the bedroom, 34% in the bathroom, 9% in the kitchen, 5% on the stairs, 4% in the living room, and the remaining 6% in other areas. This surveillance system will be used to assist the authors' study, clarifying what causes falls, and identifying and evaluating appropriate ways to prevent falls.

283 Dunn, Julie E., Rudberg, Mark A., Furner, Sylvia E., & Cassel, Christine K. (March, 1992). Mortality, disability, and falls in

older persons: The role of underlying disease and disability. *American Journal of Public Health, 82*(3), 395-400.

Data from the Longitudinal Study on Aging were analyzed to study the relationship between falls and both mortality and functional status in 4,270 respondents ages 70 and over. The methods and results of the study are discussed. The authors conclude that multiple falls in older persons increase risk of functional impairment and may indicate underlying conditions that increase risk of death.

284   Duthie, Edmund H., Jr. (November, 1989). Falls. *Medical Clinics of North America, 73*(6), 1321-1336.

The author reviews falls, which are often health hazards for the elderly patient. Fatalities are more common among the elderly: 70% of deaths from falls occur in the elderly population. Falls may be caused by environmental factors; neurologic illnesses, including dementia, drop attacks, and sensory loss; alcohol and drug use; cardiac arrhythmias; and acute illnesses such as infections, heart failure, or gastrointestinal bleeding. Physicians who treat elderly patients should be able to identify both those patients at risk as well as those who already have the problem.

285   Fiatarone, Maria A., Marks, Elizabeth C., Ryan, Nancy D., Meredith, Carol N., Lipsitz, Lewis A., & Evans, William J. (June 13, 1990). High-intensity strength training in nonagenarians: Effects on skeletal muscle. *Journal of the American Medical Association, 263*(22), 3029-3034.

This study examined the muscle weakness of the very old and its reversal by strength training. Subjects were 10 frail elderly volunteers (ages 86 to 96) living in a Boston institution. For eight weeks, the subjects performed leg exercises, lifting and lowering a controlled amount of weight with each leg. Muscle strength was greater in subjects with greater regional muscle mass and more fat-free body mass. One subject stopped training after four weeks due to strain on a previous injury. For the nine patients who finished the program, the average gain in strength was 174%. They also achieved a 9% increase in midthigh muscle area and a 48% improvement in tandem gait (walking) speed. Two subjects no longer needed a cane to walk and one became able to get out of a chair without pushing up on the arms. The authors conclude that high-resistance weight training successfully improved muscle strength and size in frail nursing home patients as old as age 96.

286   Fleming, Beth Erasmus, Wilson, Donald R., & Pendergast, David R. (October, 1991). **A portable, easily performed muscle power test and its association with falls by elderly persons.** *Archives of Physical Medicine and Rehabilitation, 72*(11), 886-889.

This article describes a study to develop and evaluate a simple, inexpensive, and safe screening test to assess falling risk in elderly persons. Subjects consisted of a control group (15 men, 8 women) of nonfallers from ages 23 to 72, and a group (19 men, 3 women) of fallers from ages 63 to 92, all of whom had fallen at least once in the past year. Subjects sat in chairs (hips and knees at 90°) with their feet over a force transducer and stood as forcefully as possible. After standing for five seconds, they sat as fast as possible. The rate of change in force for standing and sitting was calculated from data collected by computer. Of the 22 fallers, 17 were identified by a reduced rate of change in force and reduced overshoot force. The authors conclude that fallers clearly rise from a chair more slowly than non-fallers, and recommend that this type of screening could provide a foundation for further research into the causes and prevention of falls.

287   Gehlsen, Gale M., & Whaley, Mitchell H. (September, 1990). **Falls in the elderly: Part I, Gait.** *Archives of Physical Medicine and Rehabilitation, 71*(10), 735-738.

This study examined the role of gait in elderly falls. Two groups of elderly people were studied: those with a history of falls (HF), and those with no history of falls (NHF). The researchers identified several characteristics of each subject's gait by filming them walking on a treadmill: step frequency, stance time, swing time, double support time, step length, heel width, heel height, toe height, and hip, knee, and ankle angular excursion. There were 25 (7 men, 18 women) in the HF group and 30 (12 men, 18 women) in the NHF group. ANOVA analysis indicated that there was a significant (p < .05) difference between the two independent variables for heel width. The relationship between the other gait characteristics and falls in the elderly was not significant.

288   Gehlsen, Gale M., & Whaley, Mitchell H. (September, 1990). **Falls in the elderly: Part II, Balance, strength, and flexibility.** *Archives of Physical Medicine and Rehabilitation, 71*(10), 739-741.

Part II of the authors' study on elderly falls sought to determine and compare balance, muscular strength, and flexibility of two different groups of elderly people: those with a history of falls (HF) and those with no history of falls (NHF). Out of the 55 subjects (19 men, 36 women) ages 65 and over studied in Part I, 25 were HF subjects, and 30 were NHF. Static and dynamic balance was determined by a one-foot stance balance test and a backwards walking test. Hip, knee, and ankle join muscular strength were assessed on a Cybex Leg Press Dynamometer. A goniometer was used to determine hip, knee, and ankle joint flexibility. ANOVA analysis indicated a significant difference in static balance ($p <$ .001), leg strength ($p < .01$), and hip and ankle flexibility ($p < .01$) between the HF and NHF groups. The authors suggest, based on these results, that balance, leg strength, and flexibility may be factors that contribute to falls in the elderly.

289   Gerson, Lowell W., Jarjoura, David, & McCord, Gary. (January, 1989). **Risk of imbalance in elderly people with impaired hearing or vision.** *Age and Ageing, 18*(1), 31-34.

The authors evaluated the effect of impaired hearing and vision on balance in elderly people. Subjects were 977 community-dwelling elderly (ages 65 and older). Interviews with the subjects reported problems with the following: balance (21%), vision (27%), and hearing (30%). Women (63% of the sample) were 1.7 times more likely to report problems with balance than men. The authors found that impaired hearing increased the probability of reporting balance problems. Impaired vision increased the probability of reporting balance problems, but mostly in the younger old (ages 65 to 69), a finding which may be due to the elderly's accommodation to vision problems. The authors conclude that impaired vision and hearing are important risk factors for imbalance and the resulting falls and injury in this population.

290   Greenspan, Susan L., Myers, Elizabeth R., Maitland, Lauri A., Resnick, Neil M., & Hayes, Wilson C. (January 12, 1994). **Fall severity and bone mineral density as risk factors for hip fracture in ambulatory elderly.** *Journal of the American Medication Association, 271*(2), 128-133.

The purpose of this study was to determine the relative importance of fall characteristics, body habitus, and femoral bone mineral density (BMD) in predicting hip fracture in community-dwelling elderly. A total of 149 ambulatory, community-dwelling fallers (126 women, 23 men), ages 65 and over, including 72 case patients (fallers with hip fracture) and 77 control fallers (fallers with no hip fracture) were studied. The authors found significant and independent risk factors for hip fracture in both men and women related to fall characteristics and body habitus. In addition to the maintenance of bone density, reductions in fall severity using trochanteric padding or enhancement of muscle strength may provide additional strategies for prevention of hip fracture in the elderly. Each year more than 250,000 Americans fracture their hips costing $8.7 billion in medical costs and having a high risk of death, long-term loss of function, risk for institutionalization. Of these fractures, more than 90% of the patients are ages 70 and over. Low bone mass and increasing age are associated with risk. Other factors are use of long-acting benzodiazepines, impaired vision, lower limb dysfunction, neurological conditions (Parkinson's) and barbiturate use. The most commonly cited factor for increased risk of hip fracture is falling, although only 5% of falls result in a hip fracture.

291   Grisso, Jeane Ann, Kelsey, Jennifer L., Strom, Brian L., Chiu, Grace Y., Maislin, Greg, O'Brien, Linda A., Hoffman, Susie, Kaplan, Frederick, & The Northeast Hip Fracture Study Group. (May 9, 1991). Risk factors for falls as a cause of hip fracture in women. *New England Journal of Medicine, 324*(19), 1326-1331.

This case-control study examined the importance of risk factors for falls in the epidemiology of hip fracture. Case subjects were 174 women (median age 80 years) admitted with a first hip fracture to 1 of 30 hospitals in New York and Philadelphia. Controls, matched to the case patients according to age and hospital, were selected from general surgical and orthopedic surgical hospital services. Increased risks for hip fracture were associated with lower-limb dysfunction, visual impairment, previous stroke, Parkinson's disease, and use of longacting barbiturates. Of the controls, 44 (25%) had recently fallen. The case patients were more likely than controls to have fallen from a standing height or higher. Of those with hip fracture, the older patients (ages 75 and over) were less likely to have fallen on a hard surface. The authors identify the following risk factors for falls as associated with hip fracture: lower-limb dysfunction, neurologic conditions, barbiturate use, and visual impairment. Given the prevalence of these problems among the elderly, who are at highest risk, the authors recommend that programs to prevent hip fracture should include preventing falls in addition to slowing bone loss.

292   Hallbauer, Gregg Marshall. (March-April, 1993). "Sure step" — A program to strength train persons 60 or older to decrease risk of falls. *Public Health Reports, 108*(2), 172-173.

This article describes a proposed strength-training program for older adults in Tarrant County, Texas. The "Sure Step" program has the following objectives: to establish an eight-week community-based instruction and supervised strength training program, followed by a maintenance program; to use existing senior centers as training sites; to increase awareness of the risk factors for falls; and to instruct older adults in the principles of strength training. Pre- and posttests will measure the participants' gait, step height and length, and lower extremity muscle strength.

293   Hogue, Carol, C. (November, 1984). **Falls and mobility in late life: An ecological model.** *Journal of the American Geriatrics Society, 32*(11), 858-861.

Little attention has been paid to the way personal and environmental factors interact to prevent falls and improve mobility. In response, the author presents an ecological model based on the theory that behavior is a function of the person, the environment, and the interaction of the person and the environment. This model, when applied to the areas of falls and mobility, offers suggestions for methods of prevention and intervention.

294   Hornbrook, Mark C., Stevens, Victor J., & Wingfield, Darlene J. (March, 1993). **Seniors' Program for Injury Control and Education.** *Journal of the American Geriatrics Society, 41*(3), 309-314.

This article is a description of the Seniors' Program for Injury Control and Education (SPICE) which examined the effects of exercise and physical fitness on falls and related injuries in older persons. Study design was a two-group, randomized trial with two years of follow-up at the Northwest Region of Kaiser Permanente (NWKP), a large hospital-based prepaid group practice Health Maintenance Organization (HMO) in Portland, Oregon. Subjects were 1,323 community-living persons ages 65 and over enrolled in NWKP and at moderate risk of falling. A multifaceted intervention strategy used a group approach to falls and injury prevention, including moderate intensity endurance-building exercise (walking), strength and balance training, home safety improvements, and mental practice. Sessions of 20 to 25 participants were led by two nurses. The participants set their own realistic goals for exercise. The control group received usual care from the HMO. Outcome measures included health status, physical functioning, falls, and fall-related medical care use and cost. The authors suggest that if SPICE is effective, cost-effectiveness analysis will examine the relative efficiency of SPICE versus other successful interventions.

295   Jacobsen, Steven J., Goldberg, Jack, Miles, Toni P., Brody, Jacob A., Stiers, William, & Rimm, Alfred A. (1991). Seasonal variation in the incidence of hip fracture among white persons aged 65 years and older in the United States, 1984-1987. *American Journal of Epidemiology, 133*(10), 996-1004.

The authors studied data from the Health Care Financing Administration to discover whether there were seasonal variations in hip fractures. Of 621,387 hip fractures recorded from 1984 to 1987, 492,006 were suffered by elderly white women and 129,381 were suffered by elderly white men (ages 65 and over). Mean fracture rates were consistently higher in all age and gender groups during winter, and lower during summer. The authors suggest that this trend may have several causes: fewer hours of sunlight during winter months affecting those with compromised vision, decreased levels of vitamin D causing diminished bone structure during winter months, decreased body temperature in cold weather, and inclement weather (ice and snow).

296   Jech, Arlene Orhon. (January-February, 1992). Preventing falls in the elderly. *Geriatric Nursing, 34*(1), 43-44.

The author makes recommendations for a safe environment for elders cared for by relatives at home. She describes body changes that put elders at risk, including balance, vision, and thinning of bones. She recommends several home safety tips: providing proper lighting, adding handrails to stairs at the proper height, painting the first and last steps a different color or placing a knob on the banister at the first and last steps as a signal, painting outside stairs with sand-added paint, stapling telephone and electric cords to the floor or wall, eliminating throw rugs, using nonskid appliques in bathrooms, mounting handrails on the wall near the toilet, shower, and tub, wearing well-fitting shoes, and repairing walkways. She also points out that certain medications can increase the risk for falls and should be evaluated by the family physician.

297   Kerman, Marc, & Mulvihill, Michael. (November, 1990). Role of medication in falls among the elderly in a long-term care facility. *Mount Sinai Journal of Medicine, 57*(6), 343-347.

This case-control study examined the relationship between falls and drug use in elderly residents of a long-term care facility. Drug use and functional status of 57 first-time fallers were compared with those of 90 residents who had never fallen. Fallers were taking significantly more drugs than controls. Hypnotic/anxiolytics and cardiac drugs carried a twofold increase in the risk of falling. Fallers were restrained less often, were more often ambulatory, and had been at the institution for a shorter time than controls. The authors suggest that a large prospective study is needed to determine whether these results are generalizable to institutionalized elderly as a whole.

298   Kiel, Douglas P. (August, 1993). The evaluation of falls in the emergency department. *Clinics in Geriatric Medicine, 9*(3), 591-600.

Falls account for the majority of injury-related visits to an emergency department; however, the injury resulting from the fall should not be the sole focus of evaluation. This article reviews the incidence, morbidity, mortality, and causes of falls in the elderly population. Approximately one-third of community-dwelling elderly ages 75 and over fall each year, at a rate that increases to 40% in those ages 80 and over. Falls are more common in nursing home residents, where 1,600 falls per 1,000 patients has been reported. Causes of falls can be extrinsic or intrinsic, and a combination of risk factors is often found. The author outlines a clinical approach to the fall patient that includes history-taking, physical examination, and laboratory examination. Treatment involves not only treating the injury that may have resulted from the fall, but also developing a strategy to manage or eliminate the causes of the fall.

299   Klawans, Harold L., & Topel, Jordon L. (December 16, 1974). Parkinsonism as a falling sickness. *Journal of the American Medical Association, 230*(11), 1555-1557.

The authors describe 11 Parkinsonism patients (ages 64 and over), in whom loss of postural reflexes causing episodic falling was the initial and predominant manifestation of the disease. None of these patients responded to standard anticholinergic medication, but all 11 responded dramatically to amantadine or levodopa. It is important to recognize that Parkinsonian deficit can manifest itself solely or predominantly as falling.

300   Lach, Helen W., Reed, A. Thomas, Arfken, Cynthia L., Miller, J. Philip, Paige, Gary D., Birge, Stanley, J., & Peck, William A. (February, 1991). Falls in the elderly: Reliability of a classification system. *Journal of the American Geriatrics Society, 39*(2), 197-202.

This study analyzed falls among a sample of 1,358 community-dwelling elderly during a three-year period. In the first year of the study, there were 366 falls reported by 258 of the subjects, which were subsequently divided into four major categories: falls related to extrinsic factors (55%), falls related to intrinsic factors (39%), falls from a non-bipedal stance (8%), and unclassified falls (7%). The authors suggest that the classification system developed in this study provides a set of operational definitions for types of falls, and that it has proved to be a method of classifying elderly falls that is both reliable and flexible.

301   Lauritzen, J. B., Petersen, M. M., & Lund, B. (January 2, 1993). Effect of external hip protectors on hip fractures. *The Lancet, 341*(8836), 11-13.

The authors examined hip fractures among elderly residents of a nursing home in this controlled trial. Subjects were 497 women and 204 men ages 65 and over in a Copenhagen nursing home. Treatment subjects (167 women, 80 men) were given external hip protectors. During the 11 month study, there were 8 hip and 15 non-hip fractures in the treatment group, and 31 hip and 27 non-hip fractures in the control group. Nearly a third of those who fell could not explain how they fell. None of the eight treatment subjects who sustained hip fractures were wearing the external devices when they fell. Analysis of whether the hip protector was actually being worn at the time of a fall showed that no fractures occurred in the six instances when the protector was worn. The study indicates that external hip protectors can prevent hip fractures in nursing home residents.

302   Lipsitz, Lewis A., Jonsson, Palmi V., Kelley, Margaret M., & Koestner, Julia S. (1991). Causes and correlates of recurrent falls in ambulatory frail elderly. *Journals of Gerontology, 46*(4), M114-M122.

The authors evaluated 70 recurrent fallers and 56 nonfallers (mean age 87 years). Fallers were more often women, were more functionally impaired, and were taking more medications than nonfallers. Specific diseases did not distinguish fallers from nonfallers. Male and female fallers took more steps to turn 360°, could not stand up from a chair without pushing off, had a higher prevalence of antidepressant use, and had impaired position sensation. These easily obtained clinical variables characterized nearly three-quarters of ambulatory elderly nursing home residents with a history of recurrent falls.

303   Loew, François. (January, 1993). **The elderly can avoid falls.** *World Health,* 46(1), 10-11.

The author reports that up to 40% of elderly people (ages 65 and over) fall at least once a year, causing bruises and superficial injuries, and in some cases even severe injuries like fractures. Elderly falls can be caused by several things: they may be related to chronic neurological or osteoarticular diseases; cardiac or circulatory problems; the natural effects of aging on body strength, agility, and eyesight; medications; environmental hazards; or, often, a combination of two or more of these factors. As a result, the author recommends eliminating these contributing factors whenever possible as the most likely method of prevention. Precautions include getting proper diet and exercise, eliminating household hazards like loose carpets, avoiding dangerous behavior, and cutting out unnecessary medication.

304   Lord, Stephen R., Clark, Russell D., & Webster, Ian W. (1991). **Visual acuity and contrast sensitivity in relation to falls in an elderly population.** *Age and Ageing,* 20(3), 175-181.

This Australian study measured the relationship between visual acuity, contrast sensitivity, and falls among 95 elderly (mean age 83 years) residents of a hostel for the aged. Subjects were given dual-contrast letter chart tests and the Melbourne Edge Test (MET) to evaluate their level of acuity and contrast sensitivity, which was shown to decrease significantly with age. Visual acuity and contrast sensitivity were not shown to be associated with body sway when subjects stood on solid flooring, but did significantly contribute to body sway when subjects stood on a compliant surface (a six-inch thickness of foam rubber). Twenty-two subjects were unable to complete the body sway test on the foam surface because of impaired balance. Because there was a difference in contrast sensitivity between those who fell one or more times in the year of follow-up and those who did not fall, it is suggested that decreased contrast sensitivity (the ability to perceive edges like steps, cracks in the sidewalk, etc.) can be a predisposing factor in falls.

305   Lord, Stephen R., Clark, Russell, D., & Webster, Ian W.
      (December, 1991). Physiological factors associated with falls in
      an elderly population. *Journal of the American Geriatrics Society,*
      39(12), 1194-1200.
            This article describes an Australian study to examine the
      reliability of 13 sensorimotor, vestibular, and visual tests in
      predicting elderly fallers and non-fallers. There were 95 subjects,
      ages 59 to 97 (mean age 82.7 years), who were generally
      independent residents of a hostel for the aged. Tests evaluated
      visual acuity, contrast sensitivity, touch thresholds at the ankle,
      vibration sense at the knee, proprioception, vestibular stepping,
      vestibular optical stability, quadriceps strength, ankle dorsiflexion
      strength, body sway, and postural stability. During the year of
      follow-up there were 145 falls. Forty subjects reported no falls, 11
      subjects fell once, and 33 subjects fell twice or more. Discriminant
      function analysis identified several factors which significantly
      discriminated between those with one or no falls and those with
      two or more falls: proprioception in the lower limbs, visual
      contrast sensitivity, ankle dorsiflexion strength, reaction time, and
      sway with eyes closed. This procedure correctly classified 79% of
      the subjects into groups of multiple fallers or non-multiple fallers.
      The authors suggest that the physiological factors associated with
      falls by this study can be used to highlight some areas
      predisposing elderly people to falls.

306   Macdonald, John B. (August, 1985). The role of drugs in falls in
      the elderly. *Clinics in Geriatric Medicine, 1*(3), 621-636.
            This article is a brief survey of the link between drugs and
      falls. Current studies have identified risks with benzodiazepines,
      barbiturates, phenothiazines, antihypertensives, diuretics, tricyclic
      antidepressants, non-steroidal anti-inflammatory drugs (NSAID),
      antiparkinsonian drugs, alcohol, and some less common drugs.
      The more types of drugs a patient receives, the greater the
      likelihood of a fall, and combining drugs with various diseases
      also compounds the risk. The author suggests that new research
      should concentrate on naming individual drugs in larger surveys
      of falling. The use of more sophisticated statistical procedures and
      testing would also allow analysis of the specific dangers of these
      types of drug and drug/disease combinations.

307   Maki, Brian E., Holliday, Pamela J., & Topper, Anne K. (1991).
      Fear of falling and postural performance in the elderly. *Journals*
      of Gerontology, 46(4), M123-M131.

This cross-sectional study subjected elderly subjects (17 male, 83 female, ages 62 to 96) to five types of balance tests. Subjects were classified into faller or nonfaller and fear or no-fear categories to allow the influence of fear of falling and falling history to be separated in the analyses. Subjects who expressed a fear of falling did worse on some tests. The clinical scale was the only balance measure that showed a significant association with retrospective, self-reported falling history. The authors suggest that caution should be taken in interpreting balance test performance, and that studies for postural control and falling should allow for the potentially confounding influence of fear of falling.

308   Margulec, Itzhak, Librach, Gershon, & Schadel, Meir. (1970). Epidemiological study of accidents among residents of homes for the aged. *Journals of Gerontology,* 25(4), 342-346.

An epidemiological study of accidents among the elderly (ages 65 and over) was performed among a selected population of residents in homes for the aged in Israel. A protective environment was established during the years of the study, leading to the assumption that the accidents which occurred due to falls would show a greater involvement of host-linked factors than environmental ones. Accidents among 95% of all subjects were due to falls. Women were more affected, and there were more accidents in those ages 75 and over. Bone fractures were the most frequent injury, occurring mainly among women and as a result of falls. The preponderance of host-linked factors in the occurrence of accidents among the aged calls for more studies of this aspect on a international basis.

309   McIntosh, Shona J., Da Costa, David, & Kenny, Rose Anne. (January, 1993). Outcome of an integrated approach to the investigation of dizziness, falls and syncope in elderly patients referred to a 'syncope' clinic. *Age and Ageing,* 22(1), 53-58.

Syncope (fainting spells) can be associated with falls in elderly people. The authors of this article operate a syncope clinic for elderly patients with falls, dizziness, and syncope. The 65 elderly subjects (mean age 78 years) were patients at the clinic during its first six months of operation. Diagnoses (which overlapped in 25% of cases) in the subjects were cardioinhibitory carotid sinus syndrome (CSS), 5%; vasodepressor CSS, 26%; mixed CSS, 14%; orthostatic hypotension, 32%; vasodepressor vasovagal syncope, 11%; cardiac arrhythmia, 21%; epilepsy, 9%; cerebro-vascular disease, 6%; and others, 12.5%.

310 McMurdo, Marion E. T., & Gaskell, Alan. (1991). Dark adaptation and falls in the elderly. *Gerontology, 37*(4), 221-224.

This article reports the findings of a British study to determine the relationship of decreased dark adaptation to falls in elderly people. Subjects were 22 female patients (12 non-fallers, 10 fallers) in a hospital geriatric assessment ward. On dark adaptation tests, the non-faller group had a significantly higher scores on both 5-minute (p < .02) and 20-minute (p < .04) tests than the fallers. Impaired or reduced dark adaptation can leave an elderly person virtually blind temporarily when moving to a darker area from a bright room. The authors recommend the use of night lights in homes of chronic fallers to offset the influence of impaired dark adaptation.

311 Morton, Dolores. (February, 1989). Five years of fewer falls. *American Journal of Nursing, 89*(2) , 204-205.

This article describes a High Risk for Falls program at the St. John Medical Center, Tulsa, Oklahoma. The center identified the risk factors involved, then identified the patients with those risk factors. By developing a system to keep a closer watch on high-risk patients, the fall rate dropped 25% the first year, and 8% the second. A bedcheck alarm, which went off when a patient's weight was no longer in a chair or bed, allowed the center staff to attend these patients when the alarm sounded. By learning the patterns of the falls, they were able to decrease the fall rate by 60%.

312 Myers, Ann H., Baker, Susan P., Van Natta, Mark L., Abbey, Helen, & Robinson, Elizabeth C. (1991) Risk factors associated with falls and injuries among elderly institutionalized persons. *American Journal of Epidemiology, 133*, 1179-1190.

This case-control study evaluated the risk factors associated with falls and fall-related injuries in institutions for the elderly (ages 65 and over). There were 184 case subjects, and 184 control subjects matched by length of stay at a Baltimore, Maryland long-term care facility. The research included variables such as sociodemographic information, functional status, medications, and diagnoses. Risks associated with falls at all levels of care were being able to walk, being ages 90 and over, having a history of falling, and taking vasodilator medication. Among those who fell, a diagnosis of dementia and use of a diuretic were associated with fall-related injuries. The combination of these risk factors increased the relative risk of falling to 51.9. The authors recommend that clinicians identify and provide the necessary interventions for patients at highest risk.

313   Neufeld, Richard R., Tideiksaar, Rein, Yew, Elizabeth, Brooks, Frances, Young, Joyce, Browne, Gloria, & Hsu, Ming-Ann. (November, 1991). A multidisciplinary falls consultation service in a nursing home. *The Gerontologist, 31*(1), 120-123.

The authors describe the Multidisciplinary Falls Consultation Service established at a New York long-term care facility. The falls consultation team, which included members of the medical, nursing, rehabilitation, and administration departments, created an interdisciplinary approach to the prevention of falls. The program includes educational measures for staff and patients, as well as for the patients' friends and relatives. The team also established policies for the reduction of medication and restraint use where possible, and made plans to decrease environmental hazards at the facility. The authors suggest that this interdisciplinary approach to patient falls is a novel way to effectively prevent falls and fall-related injuries.

314   Nevitt, Michael C., Cummings, Steven R., Kidd, Sharon, & Black, Dennis. (May 12, 1989). Risk factors for recurrent nonsyncopal falls. *Journal of the American Medical Association, 261*(18), 2663-2668.

The authors conducted a study to determine risk factors for falls and the consequences of recurrent nonsyncopal falls in the elderly. Subjects were 325 community-dwelling elderly (ages 60 and over) who had fallen in the previous year. During the year of study, subjects reported 593 falls. Risk factors for having a single fall were few and relatively weak. The proportion of persons with two or more falls per year increased from 10% for those with none or one of the risk factors to 69% for those with four or more risk factors. The authors conclude that a complete history, tests of neuromuscular performance and vision, and a physical examination can predict, by diagnosis of risk factors, those at risk of multiple falls.

315   Ochs, Alfred L., Newberry, Janice, Lenhardt, Martin L., & Harkins, Stephen W. (1985). Neural and vestibular aging associated with falls. In James E. Birren, & K. Warner Schaie

(Eds.) *Handbook of the psychology of aging, Second edition.* (pp. 378-399). New York: Van Nostrand Reinhold Company.

This chapter reviews neurological function, balance, and falls of the elderly. Although little is known of central, vestibular, proprioceptive, and visual decrements in relationship to the tasks of walking and negotiating the physical environment, there are likely to be factors that predispose a person to falling. Knowing those factors can lead to appropriate interventions. The authors begin with a discussion of falls among the elderly in institutions and in the community and the causes of falls. The authors discuss the aging of the vestibular system and changes in the nervous system affecting equilibrium, and body sway of the elderly and their relationships to falls. They conclude that degenerative changes that occur with advanced age in the vestibular, visual, and proprioceptive sensory systems, changes in the central nervous system, and increased body sway are related to increased risk for falling in the elderly.

316　O'Loughlin, Jennifer L., Robitaille, Yvonne, Boivin, Jean-François, & Suissa, Samy. (February 1, 1993). Incidence of and risk factors for falls and injurious falls among the community-dwelling elderly. *American Journal of Epidemiology, 137*(3), 342-354.

This Canadian study analyzed the frequency of and risk factors for falls among a sample of noninstitutionalized, community-dwelling elderly (ages 65 and over). The 409 subjects (152 men, 257 women) were initially interviewed at home, and then followed-up for 18 months. During the follow-up period, 29.0% of subjects reported falls, of which 17.6% fell once, and 11.5% fell two or more times. The researchers studied several potential risk factors: sociodemographic variables, physical activity, alcohol consumption, acute and chronic health problems, dizziness, mobility, and medication. Multivariate analyses on the follow-up data found that dizziness, frequent physical activity, having days on which activities were limited because of a health problem, having trouble walking 400 meters, and having trouble bending down had statistically significant associations with increased risk of falls. Diversity of physical activities, daily alcohol consumption, spending days in bed because of a health problem, and taking heart medication were found to be protective factors.

317　Pearlman, Cindy. (February, 1994). How to avoid household falls. *Safety & Health, 149*(2), 76-79.

Falling accidents are the largest cause of preventable death in households and resulted in 6,200 deaths in 1992. The elderly are the most likely to suffer severe injury or death from household falls. This article gives a "room-by-room tour" and suggests prevention interventions for each area. For example, one way to make bathrooms safer is to use non-skid rugs. Other areas discussed are steps, kitchens, family and living rooms, and bedrooms. The author also suggests that learning the "proper" way to fall can prevent some fall-related injuries, and gives several rules and suggestions for people to follow.

318   Pentland, Brian, Jones, Patricia A., Roy, Christopher W., & Miller, J. Douglas. (July, 1986). Head injury in the elderly. *Age and Ageing, 15*(4), 193-202.

This study compared the types and causes of head injuries between 1,571 patients ages 65 and under during one year with 449 patients ages 65 and over during two one-year periods, all of whom were admitted to a head and spinal injury unit in Edinburgh, Scotland. Domestic accidents and falls were the most common causes of injuries to elderly people (75%, compared to 33% in the younger group). When severe injuries were considered alone, road traffic accidents were the most common in both groups. The elderly were more likely to have pedestrian accidents, compared with the younger group, who were more likely injured as vehicle occupants. Another common factor was alcohol: for both groups, over half of the males admitted for minor head injuries appeared to have alcohol-related injuries. Among other factors examined, both mortality and length of hospital stay were shown to increase with increasing age.

319   *Preventing falls and fractures.* (1992). Gaithersburg, MD: National Institute on Aging.

This pamphlet is designed to help elderly people avoid falls. The author gives guidelines for avoiding falls and keeping homes fall-proof.

320   Rubenstein, Laurence Z., Robbins, Alan S., Josephson, Karen R., Schulman, Barbara L., & Osterweil, Dan. (August 15, 1990). The value of assessing falls in an elderly population: A randomized clinical trial. *Annals of Internal Medicine, 113*(4), 308-316.

This study measured the effectiveness of a specialized, post-fall assessment to detect the causes and risk factors for falls, and to recommend interventions to prevent further falls. Subjects were

160 residents of a California long-term residential facility who had fallen in the past seven days. The subjects were randomly assigned to either an assessment group (n=79) or a control group (n=81). The assessment consisted of both physical and environmental examination. Based on the assessment, recommendations for prevention and therapy were given to the subject's primary physician, including factors like weakness, environmental hazards, orthostatic hypotension, drug side effects, and gait dysfunction. After two years of follow-up, the assessment group showed 26% fewer hospitalizations (p < .05) and 52% fewer hospital days (p < .01) when compared to the control group. The authors suggest that this assessment can easily identify those at risk for future falls, and as a result reduce disability and cost of injury.

321 Rubenstein, Laurence Z., Robbins, Alan S., Schulman, Barbara L., Rosado, Juan, Osterweil, Dan, & Josephson, Karen R. (1988). Falls and instability in the elderly. *Journal of the American Geriatrics Society, 36*(2), 266-278.

   This article is a detailed discussion of the epidemiology and common causes of falls and suggested diagnostic evaluations for post-fall patient follow-up, which are illustrated by two cases of elderly patients with complex fall problems typical of the elderly population. The authors also discuss three of the most important and least researched causes of falls: gait instability, muscle weakness, and environmental hazards.

322 Schnelle, John F., Mac Rae, Priscilla G., Simmons, Sandra F., Uman, Gwen, Ouslander, Joseph G., Rosenquist, Lori L., & Chang, Betty. (June, 1994). Safety assessment for the frail elderly: A comparison of restrained and unrestrained nursing home residents. *Journal of the American Geriatrics Society,* 42(6), 586-592.

   The purpose of this study was to help clinicians decide whether or not to use physical restraints with elderly patients by identifying which reversible injury risks differentiated between restrained and unrestrained nursing home residents. The researchers compared 108 physically restrained and 111 unrestrained residents of several California long-term care facilities using a safety assessment for the frail elderly (SAFE). The authors conclude that the SAFE protocol can reliably measure behavioral factors that can contribute to falls and injury in nursing homes. Because removing or changing restraints alone will not significantly improve residents' mobility, the authors recommend that restraint reduction programs be combined with interventions to decrease the influence of injury contributors measured by SAFE.

323   Shroyer, JoAnn L. (1994). **Recommendations for environmental design research correlating falls and the physical environment.** *Experimental Aging Research, 20*(4), 303-309.

Among the risk factors for falls by aging people (ages 55 and older) are environmental hazards. These risk factors fall into two groups: extrinsic and intrinsic. Extrinsic factors include floor surfaces, lighting, sensory surround and feedback, and furniture placement. Intrinsic factors include physical ability, mobility, sensory capability, illness, medications, and many others. This article lists various environmental design features, such as lighting, furnishing, and floor surfaces, which are emphasized by existing literature as possible contributors to falls. The author recommends that further research be conducted on these design features to establish concrete empirical evidence on their relationship to injury prevention, and that designers and planners should consider the impact of environmental hazards when developing plans and drawings.

324   Simoneau, Guy G., Cavanagh, Peter R., Ulbrecht, Jan S., Leibowitz, Herschel W., & Tyrrell, Richard A. (November, 1991). **The influence of visual factors on fall-related kinematic variables during stair descent by older women.** *Journals of Gerontology, 46*(6), M188-M197.

The authors studied 36 healthy women ages 55 to 70, with normal sensory feedback and visual contrast sensitivity. The subjects were selected from a panel of volunteers to study foot-stair spatial relationships while descending the middle steps of a flight of stairs. The stairs were painted black to simulate low contrast, and a high-contrast effect was produced by painting a white stripe at the edge of each stair tread. The wall panels were modifiable, so that half of the subjects were surrounded by vertical stripes and the other half by horizontal stripes as they descended. Subjects slowed their pace when their vision was blurred, and increased their foot clearance, thereby adjusting for possible errors in foot placement. The wall patterns did not make a difference. The results underscore the importance of properly fitted footwear, better contrast definition on stairs, special attention to the needs of those who wear bifocals, and the use of slip-resistant surfaces in fall prevention.

325 Simpson, Janet M., & Salkin, Sharon. (July, 1993). Are elderly people at risk of falling taught how to get up again? *Age and Ageing, 22*(4), 294-296.

Clinical experience indicates that elderly patients likely to fall down are rarely taught how to get up again, even though lying on the floor for an extended period can lead to complications such as hypothermia, dehydration and bronchopneumonia. A random sample of physiotherapists in England was studied to see how often they taught elderly patients this skill. Of the 67 usable answers, four physiotherapists (11%) and six occupational therapists (21%) indicated they would teach elderly patients how to get up after a fall.

326 Sorock, Gary S., Bush, Trudy, L., Golden, Anne L., Fried, Linda P., Breuer, Brenda, & Hale, Wiliam E. (1988). Physical activity and fracture risk in a free-living elderly cohort. *Journals of Gerontology, 43*(5), M134-M139.

This prospective study examined regular leisure-time physical activity (including recreational walking) to determine if it is associated with fracture risk. Subjects were 3,110 free-living elderly men and women in a Florida retirement community. Sixty-three percent of the cohort was female, all were white, and the average age was 73 years. Those who participated in regular physical activity had a reduced risk of fracture. Walking at least one mile three times per week appeared to offer a protective effect for both men and women. After controlling for potentially confounding variables, including body mass and selected health conditions, the result of regular physical activity on fracture incidence in men and women remained essentially unchanged. The authors conclude that regular physical activity may protect against fracture in older persons.

327 Sorock, Gary S., & Labiner, David M. (September 1, 1992). Peripheral neuromuscular dysfunction and falls in an elderly cohort. *American Journal of Epidemiology, 136*(5), 584-591.

This study tested the relationships between tests of peripheral sensory and motor functions in the lower extremities and the rate of first falls. Subjects were 169 tenants (mean age 79.8 years) of senior citizen housing in New Jersey. During a year of follow-up, 57 subjects reported at least one fall. After adjusting the fall rate for history of stroke, heart failure, emphysema, and use of walker or cane, the ratios for first falls were higher in subjects with reduced toe joint position sense, sharp-dull discrimination, and ankle strength. The presence of two or more of these factors increased the rate of falls 3.9 times. Based on the data, the authors suggest that impaired sensory and motor functions in the lower extremities play an important role in elderly falls.

328   Speechley, Mark, & Tinetti, Mary E. (January, 1991). Falls and injuries in frail and vigorous community elderly persons. *Journal of the American Geriatrics Society, 39*(1), 46-52.

The authors studied a sample of 336 community elderly to assess whether identifying different types of falls and fallers would help target injury prevention efforts more specifically to each type. The subjects were divided into three groups: frail (n=67), transitional (n=182), and vigorous (n=87). The rate of falling during the follow-up year was highest for the frail group (52%) and lowest in the vigorous group (17%), but the rate of serious injury as a result of falling was higher for the vigorous group (22%) than for the frail group (6%). When compared with frail subjects, the vigorous subjects were more likely to fall during a displacing activity (53% vs. 31%), with an environmental hazard present (53% vs. 29%), and on stairs (27% vs. 6%). The authors suggest that fall-related injuries can be serious health problems for both frail and vigorous elderly people, and that injury prevention efforts should be directed to the specific needs and differences between the fall circumstances in these two groups.

329   Stelmach, George E., Teasdale, Normand, Di Fabio, Richard P., & Phillips, Jim. (1989). Age related decline in postural control mechanisms. *International Journal of Aging and Human Development, 29*(3), 205-223.

Greater postural sway and the increased incidence of falls observed in elderly persons suggests that older individuals may be slower in detecting and correcting postural disturbances. This experiment addressed the issue by assessing postural sway and the speed of reflexive and voluntary mechanisms responsible for correcting postural disturbances in young and elderly persons. Overall, the elderly exhibited more perturbation-induced sway and were slower in voluntary reactions as opposed to reflexive. When small perturbations were given, the elderly swayed more and produced sporadic reflexive activity.

330   Stewart, Ronald B., Moore, Mary T., May, Franklin E., Marks, Ronald G., & Hale, William E. (December, 1992). Nocturia: A risk

factor for falls in the elderly. *Journal of the American Geriatrics Society, 40*(12), 1217-1220.

Nocturia is a medical condition reportedly suffered by 80% of ambulatory elderly people which requires them to arise from sleep at night to urinate. Because getting up and navigating in reduced light or darkness could be a fall risk, the authors studied a sample of ambulatory elderly in Florida. The participants, 988 women and 520 men ages 65 and over, were asked to report the number of falls they had experienced in the past year, and the number of times they got up at night to urinate. Subjects who reported nocturia were at a significantly greater risk to report falls, and the risk increased in those who reported more than three nocturia events. Based on the findings, the authors recommend that fall prevention should include prevention of nocturia.

331 Teasdale, Normand, Stelmach, George E., & Breunig, Ann. (November, 1991). Postural sway characteristics of the elderly under normal and altered visual and support surface conditions. *Journals of Gerontology, 46*(6), B238-B245.

To determine how balance is maintained, the authors compared 10 subjects in their early 20s to 18 subjects ages 70 to 80. They stood on both a normal and a foam-covered surface of a movable platform, once with their eyes open and again with them closed. Range, variability, speed and dispersion of sway were greater among the elderly subjects, and these reactions increased more among both groups when the subjects had their eyes closed. Blocking vision did not affect the older volunteers any more than the younger ones. The authors suggest that the less stable posture of the elderly is not caused by slower processing by the postural control system, but rather by a defect in the system. For elderly subjects, balance was substantially more difficult when their eyes were closed and they had to rely on input from the inner ear alone. Poor balance may also be caused by an inability to adjust to changes in two senses at the same time.

332 Tideiksaar, Rein. (1989). *Falling in old age: Its prevention and treatment.* New York: Springer Publishing Company.

This comprehensive text presents an overview of falls among the elderly. The author discusses prevalence, risk factors, medical causes of falling, and psychosocial aspects of falls. He explains how to assess and correct environmental hazards and how to assess and document fall episodes. In the appendices

Tideiksaar includes a fall diary, case studies, and descriptions of fall alarm systems.

333   **Tideiksaar, Rein. (June, 1992). Falls among the elderly: A community prevention program.** *American Journal of Public Health, 82(6),* **892-893.**

The author describes a fall prevention plan developed at the Community General Hospital in Sullivan County, New York. Because falls in older people involve an interaction of several factors, prevention requires a mixture of countermeasures and interventions to be effective. Program design included identifying a population of older persons who had had falls or related injuries and describing the extent of the problem; determining the circumstances and conditions under which these people had fallen; developing preventive interventions aimed at eliminating or ameliorating the factors identified; and finally, evaluating the effectiveness of the program.

334   **Tinetti, Mary E. (July, 1987). Factors associated with serious injury during falls by ambulatory nursing home residents.** *Journal of the American Geriatrics Society, 35(7),* **644-648.**

This study assessed factors associated with fall injuries among ambulatory nursing home residents. Subjects were 79 elderly men and women (ages 61 and over) at three intermediate care facilities in Rochester, New York. Forty-eight of the subjects fell during their first year at the facility, and 14 fallers suffered a serious injury. Subjects with lower extremity weakness were more likely to be injured than fallers without weakness (42% vs. 12% injured). On the other hand, injured fallers needed less help than noninjured fallers (14% needed help with at least two activities of daily living vs. 35%), and were less likely to be depressed than were noninjured fallers (7% vs. 38%). No injury occurred while rising from a chair. The contribution of environmental hazards was not well defined. The only acute factor distinguishing noninjurious from injurious falls was a recent previous fall (30% vs. 0%). The finding that injured fallers tend to be more independent, yet have greater lower extremity weakness, than noninjured fallers suggests that both components of injury (force of impact and protective responses of the faller) may contribute to risk of injury during a fall. The author suggests that if predictive characteristics of the injury-prone faller, or the fall, can be identified, preventive strategies could be targeted at high-risk groups.

335 Tinetti, Mary E., Liu, Wen-Liang, & Claus, Elizabeth B. (January 6, 1993). **Predictors and prognosis of inability to get up after falls among elderly persons.** *Journal of the American Medical Association, 269*(1), 65-70.

This study examined the factors that predict an elderly person's ability to get up after falling, and the effect that inability to get up can have on the resulting consequences of falling. Subjects were 1,103 Connecticut residents ages 72 and over. During the two-year follow-up, subjects reported 596 non-injurious falls. In 220 of these fall incidents, the subject was unable to get up without assistance. Of 313 non-injured fallers, 148 (47%) reported not being able to get up after at least one fall. Several risk factors were significantly associated (in comparison with non-fallers) with inability to get up, including being among ages 80 and over, depression, and poor balance and gait. Among fallers, older age and poor balance and gait were marginally associated with inability to get up. Compared with fallers who were able to get up, fallers unable to get up were more likely to die, to be hospitalized, and to suffer at least three days of impaired daily living activities. The authors suggest that the frequency of inability to get up and the morbidity associated with it demonstrate a need for prevention and treatment efforts.

336 Tinetti, Mary E., Richman, Donna, & Powell, Lynda. (1990). **Falls efficacy as a measure of fear of falling.** *Journals of Gerontology, 45*(6), P239-P243.

The authors developed a test measure called the Falls Efficacy Scale (FES) on the definition of fear as "low perceived self-efficacy at avoiding falls during essential, nonhazardous activities of daily living." The reliability and validity of the FES were assessed. The FES showed good test-retest reliability. Subjects who reported avoiding activities because of fear of falling had higher FES scores, representing lower self-confidence, than subjects not reporting fear of falling. It was found that the FES appears to be a reliable and valid method for measuring fear of falling. This instrument may be useful in assessing the independent contribution of fear of falling to functional decline and falls among elderly people.

337 Tinetti, Mary E., & Speechley, Mark. (April 20, 1989). **Prevention of falls among the elderly.** *The New England Journal of Medicine, 320*(16), 1055-1059.

This article reviews the subject of falls among the elderly, and discusses four major categories of risk factors for falls: chronic, short-term, activity-related, and environmental. Prevention of falls involves careful assessment and modification of these predisposing disabilities and risk factors. The authors suggest that identifying those patients at risk for falls and intervening to decrease that risk should be a high priority for health professionals.

338   Tinetti, Mary E., Speechley, Mark, & Ginter, Sandra F. (December 29, 1988). Risk factors for falls among elderly persons living in the community. *The New England Journal of Medicine, 319*(26), 1701-1707.

The authors studied risk factors for falling in a one-year prospective investigation. Subjects were 336 community-dwelling elderly (ages 75 and older). All subjects were assessed by a detailed clinical evaluation that included standardized measures of mental status, strength, reflexes, balance, and gait. In addition, home environmental hazards were identified. Falls and their circumstances were identified during bimonthly telephone calls. During a year of follow-up, 108 subjects (32%) fell at least once. Of these, 24% had serious injuries and 6% had fractures. Predisposing factors for falls were identified in linear-logistic models: sedative use, cognitive impairment, disability of the lower extremities, palmomental reflex, abnormalities of balance and gait, and foot problems. Risk of falling increased linearly with the number of risk factors, from 8% with none to 78% with four or more (p < .0001). About 10% of the falls occurred during acute illness, 5% during hazardous activity, and 44% in the presence of environmental hazards. The authors conclude that falls among community-dwelling elderly are common, and that a simple clinical assessment can identify those at greatest risk.

339   Urton, Maxine M. (March-April, 1991). A community home inspection approach to preventing falls among the elderly. *Public Health Reports, 106*(2), 192-195.

This article describes a comprehensive program to prevent falls among the elderly in Wilmington, Ohio, which incorporates the use of the community senior citizens' center, the local college, fire department, local radio stations and newspapers, community churches, local merchants, educators, and the medical community. Extrinsic factors previously linked to falls are identified by home inspections. The "Fixer-Up-Team," composed of college students and community volunteers, is assigned to fix any unsafe condition found by the inspection team. Local merchants and lumber yards donate materials to make needed repairs. Active senior citizens are also trained as part of the inspection team, allowing this program to be self-perpetuating. Compared to the national prevalence rates, this program is designed show a decrease in injuries caused by falls in the homes of the participants of this program.

340 Vetter, Norman J., Lewis, Peter A., & Ford, Diane. (April 4, 1992). Can health visitors prevent fractures in elderly people? *British Medical Journal, 304*(6831), 888-890.

This randomized, controlled trial assessed whether intervention by a health visitor could reduce the number of fractures, over a four-year period in those ages 70 and over. Subjects were 674 (350 intervention, 324 control) patients from a general practice in a British market town. The intervention group was allocated to the care of a health visitor with four objectives: assessment and correction of nutritional deficiencies, including reducing smoking and alcohol intake; assessment and referral of medical conditions such as heart block or inappropriate medication; assessment and correction of environmental hazards in the home, such as poor lighting; and improvement of fitness. The intervention continued for four years. The incidence of fractures was 5% (16/350) in the intervention group and 4% (14/324) in the control group (difference not significant). The authors conclude that a health visitor using simple preventive measures had no effect on the incidence of fractures.

341 Wagner, Edward H., LaCroix, Andrea Z., Grothaus, Lou, Leveille, Suzanne G., Hecht, Julia A., Artz, Karen, Odle, Kristine, & Buchner, David M. (November, 1994). Preventing disability and falls in older adults: A population-based randomized trial. *American Journal of Public Health, 84*(11), 1800-1806.

This article presents the results of a randomized controlled trial testing a multicomponent intervention program. Subjects were a random sample of health maintenance organization enrollees ages 65 and over. The 1,559 subjects were randomly divided into three groups: a nurse assessment visit and follow-up interventions targeting risk factors for disability (group one, n = 635); a general health promotion nurse visit (group two, n=607), and usual care (group three, n=607). Data collection consisted of a baseline and two annual follow-up surveys. The risk factors included in the screening were physical inactivity, excessive use of alcohol, hazards in the home, use of high-risk prescription drugs, and uncorrected hearing or visual impairments. Group one subjects attended a 60- to 90-minute visit with a trained nurse/educator. During the visit, the nurse reviewed risk factors that had been assessed on the baseline questionnaire, performed screening for hearing and blood pressure, and developed a tailored follow-up intervention plan to address any identified risk factors, and to encourage the subjects to increase physical and social activities. Results after one year found that group one subjects reported a significantly lower incidence of declining functional status and a significantly lower incidence of falls than group three subjects. Group two subjects had intermediate levels of most outcomes. After two years of follow-up, the differences narrowed. The authors conclude that the one-time intervention appears to have short-term health benefits.

342   Walker, J. Elizabeth, & Howland, Jonathan. (February, 1991). Falls and fear of falling among elderly persons living in the community: Occupational therapy interventions. *American Journal of Occupational Therapy, 45*(2), 119-122.

The authors of this article studied the incidence of falls and the prevalence, intensity and covariates of fear of falling in a sample of 115 elderly residents of a Massachusetts housing development. The mean age of subjects was 78 years. In interviews, 53% of the subjects reported falling in recent years, and 32% reported having a fall in the last year. On a scale of common fears, fear of falling ranked first. The authors suggest the following prevention interventions: 1. educating elderly people about the risk factors for and misconceptions about falls; 2. helping elderly patients eliminate environmental hazards; 3. teaching patients to avoid risky behaviors; 4. teaching patients to ask for help instead of placing themselves at risk; and 5. helping patients maintain or improve their level of physical fitness.

343   Wallace, Robert B., Ross, Jo Ellen, Huston, Jeffrey C., Kundel, Carolyn, & Woodworth, George. (March, 1993). Iowa FICSIT trial: The feasibility of elderly wearing a hip joint protective garment to reduce hip fractures. *Journal of the American Geriatrics Society, 41*(3), 338-340.

The Iowa FICSIT site is investigating passive protection during falls by the use of hip pads. The pad is designed to disperse the energy created by a fall. The authors want to determine if the elderly will wear hip pads for the majority of their waking hours.

Thirty subjects are being recruited from each of six high-risk elderly populations. Factors identifying these at-risk groups include previous hip fracture, Parkinson's disease, post-stroke rehabilitation, dementia, and history of falls. Run-in period, graduated implementation, tailoring of wearing times, and self-report of compliance will be used to facilitate compliance with the study. Outcome measures include the rates of compliance and the number of fall-related injuries.

344 Whipple, Robert H., Wolfson, Leslie I., & Amerman, Paula. (January, 1987). The relationship of knee and ankle weakness to falls in nursing home residents: An isokinetic study. *Journal of the American Geriatrics Society, 35*(1), 13-20.

This study compared the strength of the knees and ankles of a group of nursing home residents with a history of falls (n=17) to age- and gender-matched controls (n=17). The authors recorded peak torque and power at two limb velocities on a Cybex II Isokinetic dynamometer for four muscle groups: knee extensors, knee flexors, ankle plantar flexors and ankle dorsiflexors. Peak torque and power in fallers were significantly lower for all four muscle groups in comparison to controls. Differences were greatest in ankle measurements. Although power in fallers was significantly lower at the higher velocity in both joints, the decrease was most prominent in the ankles. Dorsiflexion power production in fallers was the most affected (7.5 times less than the control value). The authors conclude that at the higher, more functional limb velocities, ankle weakness appears to be an important factor underlying poor balance.

345 Wickham, C., Cooper, C., Margetts, B. M., & Barker, D. J. P. (January, 1989). Muscle strength, activity, housing and the risk of falls in elderly people. *Age and Ageing, 18*(1), 47-51.

The authors conducted a national survey in England, Wales, and Scotland to assess fall risks in elderly people. Subjects were 983 randomly selected community-dwelling elderly (ages 65 and over). Survey results were analyzed by multiple logistic regression, associating history of one or more falls with several social and physical variables identified by the survey. Subjects who had fallen one or more times were found to have less grip strength and mobility. They were also more likely to use non-phenothiazine tranquilizers, to live alone, to have recently lost weight, or to be physically disabled. Residential factors not associated with these physical factors were also strongly related to falls. The authors suggest that this relationship is caused by housing differences, like homes without indoor lavatories, old homes, and homes with inadequate heat.

346   Wild, Deidre, Nayak, U. S. L., & Isaacs, B. (January 24, 1981). How dangerous are falls in old people at home? *British Medical Journal, 282,* 266-271.

The authors surveyed subjects in six general practices in Birmingham, England, who fell in their own homes. Subjects were 125 elderly (ages 65 and over). Three had fractured their femurs and 15 had other fractures; most of the rest suffered only trivial injuries. One-quarter of these patients died within one year of the fall, five times as many as in an age- and gender-matched control group. Twenty lay on the floor for more than one hour; none were known to have suffered hypothermia. Of these, half died within six months of the fall. Factors associated with mortality from falls were impaired mobility, abnormal balance, and a disturbed pattern of gait. The authors conclude that falls at home among the elderly often indicate the presence of severe ill health.

347   Wolf-Klein, Gisele P., Silverstone, Felix A., Basavaraju, Nerlige, Foley, Conn J., Pascaru, Adina, & Ma, Pi-Huai. (September, 1988). Prevention of falls in the elderly population. *Archives of Physical Medicine and Rehabilitation, 69,* 689-691.

This article describes a falls clinic established at a New York geriatric care center. The coordinated expertise of a geriatrician, neurologist, cardiologist, and physiatrist were combined with resources in audiology, ophthalmology, and podiatry. Subjects were 36 elderly patients (24 women, mean age 79.6 years; 12 men, mean age 75.4 years). Previous to the falls clinic, subjects had sustained a total of 36 falls resulting in 13 fractures and seven soft-tissue injuries. Falls were a daily occurrence for three patients, weekly for five patients, monthly for 10, semiannually for 14, and yearly for four patients. As the team identified potential etiologic factors for falls such as medication, cardiac arrhythmias, hypotension, and visual impairment, medical management was instituted to correct the problem. Interventions included changes in medication, correction of visual problems, and safe ambulation and transfer instruction. Treatment included home visits by an occupational therapist to assess and adapt the environment, as well as educating patients, families, and caregivers regarding appropriate equipment and precautions. For some, the principal intervention was the evaluation process, with its focus on falls and prevention. The history taken for each patient included the total number of falls sustained, frequency of falls, usual time of falls, location of falls, injury sustained, medical services required, existence of fear of falling, and change in activities since the onset of falls. A one-year follow-up showed that 77% of the patients experienced no further falls. The authors suggest that falls are a multidisciplinary issue and recommend a team approach for successful management.

348   Work, Janis A. (November, 1989). Strength training: A bridge to independence for the elderly. *The Physician and Sportsmedicine,* 17(11), 134-140.

The common concept of old age as inevitable, increasing frailty and loss of physical abilities is not necessarily true, according to recent research about strength training for elderly people. There are few risks and numerous benefits to be derived from muscle group strength training. A good program involves the performance of graded exercise to develop muscle strength while increasing flexibility through low-impact aerobic exercise. Many new weight machines significantly decrease the risk for the elderly. Some of the new safety features even include mechanisms that protect the elderly from loss of balance or damage to the lower back. The machines also have better handgrips and are designed so that light weights can be used initially and increased in small increments. The social context of strength training is also beneficial for elderly people.

349   Zylke, Jody W. (April 18, 1990). As nation grows older, falls become greater source of fear, injury, death. *Journal of the American Medical Association,* 263(15), 2021.

Despite the frequency with which falls occur in the elderly and the significant morbidity and mortality they produce, relatively little is known about how and why people fall and even less is known about how to prevent them. Researchers from a number of fields are starting to investigate ways to prevent falls and consequent injures in the elderly. The author gives statistics about occurrence of falls and injury rates and discusses factors that produce a fall.

350   Zylke, Jody W. (April 18, 1990). Research focuses not only on where, why, how of falls, but also on preventing them. *Journal of the American Medical Association,* 263(15), 2022-2023.

The author discusses different approaches to fall prevention, such as SAFE (Study to Assess Falls Among the Elderly), being conducted by the Unintentional Injuries Branch at the Centers for Disease Control in Atlanta, Georgia, a National Research Council report released in February 1990 entitled "Human Factors Research Needs for an Aging Population," the Fall-Safe intervention systems, and the use of active and passive airbags to reduce the severity of injury from falls.

8

Food Poisoning

The United States Department of Agriculture estimates that over seven million cases of food poisoning (also referred to as foodborne illness) requiring medical treatment occur each year. Public health officials estimate the actual number of cases to be closer to 80 million annually. The elderly comprise one of the most at-risk populations for serious results from these happenings and are the most likely group to suffer fatalities. The most common causes are food left at room temperature for too long a period of time, poor hygiene, and improper food handling. The articles in this chapter discuss prevalence issues, hazards, and prevention. Some of the articles focus on specific types of food poisoning, symptoms of food poisoning, and treatment.

351 Bean, Nancy H., Griffin, Patricia M., Goulding, Joy S., & Ivey, Cecile B. (March, 1990). Foodborne disease outbreaks, 5-year summary, 1983-1987. *Morbidity and Mortality Weekly Report, 39*(SS-1), 15-57.

   This article is a report of foodborne disease outbreaks, defined here as incidents involving two or more people experiencing similar illness directly related to food. During 1983 to 1987, 2,397 outbreaks were reported, representing a total of 91,678 cases of food poisoning. In situations with confirmed causes (38% of total outbreaks studied), bacterial agents were responsible for 66% of outbreaks, and 92% of cases. Chemical agents caused 26% of outbreaks, and 2% of cases; parasites caused 4% of outbreaks and less than 1% of cases; and viral agents caused 5% of outbreaks, and 5% of cases. The fact that less than half of the outbreaks had confirmed etiologies suggests that methods of investigation should be improved. The authors conclude that the disparity between the number of outbreaks compared to the number of actual cases in each cause category indicates that both figures should be included in any study of food poisoning.

352   **Deli items may dish up dose of listeria. (July-August, 1992).** *FDA Consumer, 26*(6), 9-13.

This article describes Listeria monocytogenes, a group of foodborne bacteria that may cause little or no illness in healthy people, but can present a significant risk to the elderly, those with impaired immune systems, pregnant women, and newborns. Risk for listeriosis can be reduced by handling food properly, avoiding soft deli cheeses, and reheating leftover or ready-to-eat foods (such as hot dogs or deli cold cuts) before eating. The article gives examples of listeriosis outbreaks, practical food-handling tips, and other available information, as well as discussing Food and Drug Administration efforts to control listeria in food products.

353   **Harning, Abigail T. (August, 1992). Stirring up trouble: Food-related emergencies.** *Journal of Emergency Medical Services, 17*(8), 24-30; 79-88.

This article reviews the nature, risks, and management of food-related emergencies. These emergencies are divided into three categories: acute gastroenteritis caused by bacteria or parasite infection, neurological syndromes caused by bacteria infection, and allergic reactions to food. The author describes the effects and symptoms of the agents involved in each category, and gives directions for emergency treatment of each case. Prevention of illness and death from food poisoning may be accomplished by handling food properly to reduce the risk of emergencies, and by promptly reporting and treating emergencies when they occur.

354   **Labbé, Ronald G. (July-August, 1991). Clostridium perfringens.** *Journal of the Association of Official Analytical Chemists, 74*(4), 711-714.

Clostridium perfringens is a common cause of bacterial food poisoning in humans primarily associated with meat and poultry prepared in restaurants. This bacteria is commonly found in food service establishments and institutional settings because it can survive the cooking process and continue to grow at relatively high temperatures, especially when large quantities of food are prepared in advance of serving and left on low heat to keep warm. Infection with this bacteria may cause severe diarrhea and abdominal pain, as well as nausea, fever, and vomiting. Death is not common, except among those who are institutionalized or in poor health, and particularly among the elderly. Because this type of food poisoning can be prevented by proper food handling, the author suggests that previously cooked food should be refrigerated promptly, and then properly reheated before serving.

355   Levine, William C., Smart, Joanne F., Archer, Douglas L., Bean, Nancy H., & Tauxe, Robert V. (October 16, 1991). Foodborne disease outbreaks in nursing homes, 1975 through 1987. *Journal of the American Medical Association, 266*(15), 2105-2109.

This study used Centers for Disease Control data to examine the epidemiology of food poisoning outbreaks in nursing homes. During 1975 to 1987, 26 states reported 115 outbreaks of food poisoning in nursing homes that caused illness for 4,944 persons, hospitalization for 213, and death for 51. These outbreaks represented 2% of all reported foodborne disease outbreaks and 19% of outbreak- associated deaths in this period. Of the 52 outbreaks with a confirmed cause, Salmonella was the most common, accounting for 52% of outbreaks and 81% of deaths, followed by staphylococcal foodborne disease, accounting for 23% of outbreaks and 0.4% of deaths. The authors suggest that, because the elderly are at high risk for illness and death from food poisoning, nursing homes should practice careful food handling, preparation, and storage procedures; teach food handlers how to handle and prepare food safely; and develop programs to rapidly detect and control outbreaks when they occur.

356   Outbreak of Salmonella enteritidis infection associated with consumption of raw shell eggs (May 29, 1992). *Morbidity and Mortality Weekly Report, 41*(21), 369-372.

This article describes an outbreak of Salmonella poisoning at a restaurant that was traced to salad dressing made from infected eggs. Fifteen diners became ill within three days after eating at the restaurant, and 14 had eaten Caesar salad. The salad dressing and ingredients (including eggs) were not available for analysis, but Salmonella enteritidis was detected in some eggs delivered by the same supplier. Salmonella enteritidis is the most commonly reported cause of salmonella poisoning in the United States. Raw or uncooked eggs are the most likely source of infection.

Salmonella poisoning can be fatal to young children, to the elderly, and to people with impaired immune systems.

357   Ryan, Caroline A., Tauxe, Robert V., Hosek, Gary W., Wells, Joy G., Stoesz, Paul A., McFadden, Harry W., Jr., Smith, Philip W., Wright, Gregg F., & Blake, Paul A. (October, 1986). Escherichia coli O157:H7 diarrhea in a nursing home: Clinical, epidemiological, and pathological findings. *Journal of Infectious Diseases, 154*(4), 631-638.

This article describes an outbreak of Escherichia coli (E. coli) illness at a nursing home. Among the 101 residents, there were 19 confirmed, 9 probable, and 6 possible cases of E. coli, which resulted in diarrhea, colitis, kidney disorders, and four deaths. None of the 84 staff members reported any illness during the outbreak. The investigation revealed that hamburger patties served at one meal were the most likely cause of the illness. The four deaths included one patient with clostridium perfringens (another foodborne bacteria) infection, one patient who experienced fluid management complications, and two patients who developed a high fever.

358   Telzak, Edward E., Budnick, Lawrence D., Greenberg, Michele S. Zweig, Blum, Steve, Shayegani, Mehdi, Benson, Charles E., & Schultz, Stephen. (August 9, 1990). A nosocomial outbreak of Salmonella enteritidis infection due to the consumption of raw eggs. *New England Journal of Medicine, 323*(6), 394-398.

This study examined an outbreak of Salmonella enteritidis infection at a New York City hospital. Illness was seen in 404 (42%) of the patients at the hospital, and nine patients (mean age 77.5 years) died. Investigation revealed that the cause of infection was raw eggs used to make mayonnaise for patients on low-sodium diets. As a result of this outbreak, the New York State Department of Health recommended that health care facilities eliminate the use of raw or undercooked eggs for high-risk patients: the elderly, the institutionalized, and those with impaired immune systems.

359   Wilkinson, P. J., Dart, S. P., & Hadlington, C. J. (June, 1991). Cook-chill, cook-freeze, cook-hold, *sous vide*: Risks for hospital patients. *Journal of Hospital Infection, 18*(Supplement A), 222-229.

The authors describe methods of food handling that may put hospital patients at risk for food poisoning. In institutional settings, the need for large quantities of food prepared in advance and kept warm, and the use of reheated leftovers for economical reasons can put the institutionalized, elderly, or hospitalized patient at considerable risk for food-related illness. The authors describe current techniques for food handling, preparation, and storage, comparing them with current British and American government regulations and the specific characteristics of common foodborne disease.

9

Hypothermia and Hyperthermia

B̲oth hypothermia and hyperthermia are more common among elderly populations than other segments of the United States population. Hypothermia is one of the leading causes of death among elderly people in the United States. Hyperthermia, while affecting fewer people than extreme cold, can often be fatal to an elderly person. This chapter lists articles which discuss the prevalence of these injuries and describe risk factors, hazardous situations, and prevention techniques.

360 *Accidental hypothermia.* (October, 1993). Bethesda, MD: National Institute on Aging.
   This pamphlet describes the danger that elderly people face from hypothermia. Signs of hypothermia include confusion or sleepiness, slowed speech, weak pulse, signs that a person has been in a cold place, and poor control over body movement. The only way to diagnose hypothermia is with a thermometer that can register temperatures below 94°F. The pamphlet gives safety tips to protect older people from the cold, and to prevent hypothermia in even mild temperatures.

361 Albiin, Nils, & Eriksson, Anders. (1984). Fatal accidental hypothermia and alcohol. *Alcohol & Alcoholism, 19*(1), 13-22.
   The authors studied 51 fatal cases of hypothermia in Sweden. Victims were mostly male, and most cases of hypothermia occurred during winter months. Approximately two-

thirds of the victims were under the influence of alcohol. At least half of the victims could be considered alcoholics. The authors suggest that this series of cases illustrates the two main groups of hypothermia sufferers: elderly people, most of whom are under the influence of alcohol, who accounted for two-thirds of cases in this study; and younger, sober people participating in cold-weather sports like skiing or hiking.

362   Avery, Carol E., & Pestle, Ruth E. (August, 1987). Hypothermia and the elderly: Perceptions and behaviors. *The Gerontologist,* 27(4), 523-526.

The authors interviewed 381 low-income Florida residents ages 65 and older to determine their awareness of hypothermia, their perceptions of their environment, and the techniques they used to keep warm. Only 1 in 10 of the subjects was familiar with the term or considered him or herself at risk, and even fewer knew how to recognize, prevent, or treat hypothermia. Data gained from the interviews showed that many of the subjects were potentially at risk for hypothermia due to prescribed medications, caffeine or alcohol intake, smoking, homes with inadequate heating or insulation, and lack of warm clothing or bedding. The authors conclude that educational programs about hypothermia should be initiated by those who work with the elderly, even in warmer climates that are not usually considered high-risk areas.

363   Brody, Gerald M. (February, 1994). Hyperthermia and hypothermia in the elderly. *Clinics in Geriatric Medicine, 10*(1), 213-229.

Elderly people are at higher risk for hyperthermia and hypothermia than younger people due to decreased ability to sense a warm environment, decreased temperature at which they begin to sweat, and decreased vasodilator responses to heat. Chronic disease and multiple medications may also decrease an elderly person's ability to regulate body heat. Hyperthermia and hypothermia carry a high mortality rate in the older populations. The author describes in detail the physiological effects of these thermoregulatory problems, and describes the best course of treatment for each.

364   Bross, Michael H., Nash, Binford T., Jr., & Carlton, Frederick B., Jr. (August, 1994). Heat emergencies. *American Family Physician,* 50(2), 389-396.

Heat emergencies like heat exhaustion and heatstroke occur when the body cannot adequately dissipate heat. Risks for these emergencies include dehydration, inappropriate heavy clothing, certain medications, prolonged exertion, poor muscle conditioning, lack of acclimation, obesity, sleep deprivation, alcoholism, poor living conditions, chronic disease, impaired mobility, and the physiologic decline that accompanies aging. As a result, the elderly and those who perform rigorous tasks outdoors are at particular risk. The authors recommend that physicians stress three things to promote safe activity and prevent heat emergencies: heat acclimation (gradually increasing heat exposure over a period of 10 to 14 days), proper hydration (drinking at least eight ounces of water before heat exposure and during intense exertion), and proper clothing (light, single-layer clothing that allows body sweat to evaporate).

365   Celestino, Frank S., Van Noord, Glenn R., & Miraglia, Colleen P. (March, 1988). Accidental hypothermia in the elderly. *Journal of Family Practice, 26*(3), 259-267.
       This article begins with an overview of the clinical definitions and signs of the different levels of hypothermia. After describing the case of an elderly hypothermia victim, the authors describe the epidemiology, predisposing factors, and complications of hypothermia in elderly people. Risk of hypothermia is highest among the very old (ages 75 and older) and those with chronic diseases. Factors that predispose the elderly to hypothermia include decreased physiological responses to temperature, diminished muscle mass and fat, exposure, poor living conditions, medications, alcohol, nutritional deficiencies, metabolic problems, and cardiovascular diseases. Complications may include pneumonia, aspiration, shock, congestive heart failure, arrhythmias, stroke, or seizures. The authors recommend that physicians ask their patients about their living conditions, diet, exercise, drugs, and alcohol intake to identify those at risk, and that they closely monitor hypothermia-related conditions and diseases during colder months.

366   Collins, K. J. (December, 1987). Effects of cold on old people. *British Journal of Hospital Medicine, 38*(6), 506-514.
       This article examines the nature of cold weather mortality among the elderly people in Britain. The elderly are at greater risk from environmental cold because of a decreased ability to regulate body temperature and changes in sensory perception. British

statistics indicate that elderly deaths from hypothermia are small compared to the high seasonal morbidity and mortality from cardiovascular and respiratory diseases during winters in Britain.

367   **Collins, Kenneth. (February, 1988). Hypothermia in the elderly. *Health Visitor, 61*(2), 50-51.**

Statistics from the United States and Britain show that hypothermia in the overall population occurs most often in the coldest winter months. In the elderly, however, there appears to be a consistent pattern of hypothermia throughout the year. According to the author, this indicates that hypothermia in the elderly population is not exclusively induced by exposure to cold, but that it may also be caused by predisposing factors like malnutrition, chronic illness, alcohol, and medication. The author suggests that improving indoor climate, providing adequate clothing, and installing warning systems in nursing facilities may help prevent hypothermia.

368   **Darowski, A., Najim, Z., Weinberg, J. R., & Guz, A. (March, 1991). Hypothermia and infection in elderly patients admitted to hospital. *Age and Ageing,* 20(2), 100-106.**

This study assessed factors that contributed to cases of hypothermia in a British hospital. Subjects were 25 elderly patients (ages 63 and over). Four factors were associated with hypothermia in these cases: extreme age, severe illness (usually infection) or medication, living alone, and cold weather. These factors were not necessarily present in all cases. For instance, 44% of the cases studied were admitted to the hospital from warm environments, and 12% of the cases were developed during warm weather. The authors conclude that the elderly are susceptible to hypothermia due to impaired heat regulation, which may be caused by medication, infection, or a combination of factors.

369   **Halle, Alan, & Repasy, Andrew. (May 30, 1987). Classic heatstroke: A serious challenge for the elderly. *Hospital Practice,* 22(5A), 26-35.**

Classic (non-exertional) heatstroke is more common among the elderly and the socially disadvantaged than in other segments of the population. Classic heatstroke is caused by a failure of thermoregulation in a warm environment. In the elderly, the problem is exacerbated by age-related impaired heat loss, so that body temperatures rise even with minor increases in heat. Drugs like diuretics, antihistamines, and vasoconstrictors that are often taken by elderly people can amplify the effects of heat. Physical conditions often experienced by the elderly, like congestive heart failure and diabetes mellitus, can also compound heat-related risk. The authors suggest that paying attention to diet and health risks, moving to cooler environments and limiting physical activity during especially hot weather, acclimatizing older people to warmer temperatures, and educating health care workers may be effective methods of hyperthermia prevention.

370   Harchelroad, Fred. (August, 1993). **Acute thermoregulatory disorders.** *Clinics in Geriatric Medicine, 9*(3), 621-639.

Most clinicians agree that geriatric patients with thermoregulatory disorders have higher rates of morbidity and mortality than normal geriatric patients or nongeriatric patients as a whole. As a result, thermoregulatory disorders must be diagnosed early and managed in a timely manner. This article explains the process of thermoregulation in the human body, and the ways that normal aging decreases the ability of the body to regulate heat. The author also describes the common causes and treatments for hypothermia and hyperthermia in geriatric patients.

371   **Heat-associated mortality—New York City.** (July 27, 1984). *Morbidity and Mortality Weekly Report, 33*(29), 430-432.

The death rate in New York City during a June, 1984 heat wave increased 35% over the average rate for the previous four weeks. The greatest rate increase occurred in those ages 75 and over. Among those aged 75 to 84, death rates rose 39% for men, and 66% for women. For those ages 85 and over, increases were 15% for men, and 55% for women. This increased death rate was almost exclusively among persons living at home. Among those ages 65 and over, there was a 150% increase in the number of deaths occurring at home. According to the report, these data suggest that noninstitutionalized elderly, particularly elderly women, are at the highest risk of heat-associated death.

372   **Heat-related deaths—Philadelphia and United States, 1993-1994.** (July 1, 1994). *Morbidity and Mortality Weekly Report, 43*(25), 453-455.

This article reports recent heat-related mortality statistics in the United States. During a heat wave in Philadelphia, Pennsylvania, 118 people died of heat-related causes from July 6-14, 1993. Heat was also a factor in the deaths of 5,224 people in the US during 1979 to 1991. Those at increased risk for heat-related illness and death are the very young, the elderly, and those who are physically active in hot environments. Heat-related illness may also be compounded by dehydration due to certain medications, chronic illness, or consumption of alcohol. Because air conditioning reduces the risk of heat-related problems, poverty is also a risk factor. Taking advantage of air conditioned environments, cooling the body, drinking plenty of fluids, and restricting exercise to cooler parts of the day can reduce the risk for heat-related illness.

373   *Hyperthermia: A hot weather hazard for older people.* (August, 1989). Bethesda, MD: National Institute on Aging.

This pamphlet describes the risks associated with heat for older adults. In addition to describing the causes and risk factors for heat-related illness, the pamphlet also discusses treatment and prevention techniques.

374   **Illness and death due to environmental heat—Georgia and St. Louis, Missouri, 1983. (June 15, 1984).** *Morbidity and Mortality Weekly Report, 33*(23), 325-326.

Heatstroke is a condition characterized by a substantial elevation in core body temperature, generally to 40.5°C (105°F) or higher, with temperatures above 43.3°C (110°F) not uncommon. Heatstroke is often fatal, even when treated. Age-specific heatstroke rates for the summer of 1983 in St. Louis, Missouri and Georgia reveal that the elderly have a higher predisposition to heatstroke, a finding that is consistent with previous research. In St. Louis, 65.7% of heat-related deaths occurred in those ages 60 and over. In Georgia, the elderly accounted for 57% of heat-related deaths. Heatstroke rates are also higher among alcoholics. During heat waves, heatstroke prevention efforts should focus on those at greatest risk (the poor, elderly, or chronically ill). Those at risk should be advised to reduce physical activity, consume extra liquids, and, if possible, seek shelter in an air-conditioned environment for at least part of the day.

375   **Jones, T. Stephen, Liang, Arthur P., Kilbourne, Edwin M., Griffin, Marie R., Patriarca, Peter A., Wassilak, Steven G. Fite, Mullan, Robert J., Herrick, Robert F., Donnell, H. Denny, Choi, Keewhan, & Thacker, Stephen B.** (June 25, 1982). Morbidity and mortality associated with the July 1980 heat wave in St. Louis and Kansas City, Mo. *Journal of the American Medical Association, 247*(24), 3327-3331.

This study examined the rates of morbidity and mortality during the 1980 heat wave in St. Louis and Kansas City, Missouri. Heat-related illnesses and deaths were identified by reviewing the death certificates and hospital records in the two cities. Data from the July, 1980 heat wave were compared with data from July, 1978 and 1979, when there were no heat waves. Deaths by all causes in July, 1980 increased by 57% and 64% in St. Louis and Kansas City, respectively, but only 10% in the predominantly rural areas of Missouri. Approximately 1 in 1,000 residents of the two cities was hospitalized for or died of heat-related illness. Incidence rates (per 100,000) of heatstroke were 26.5 for St. Louis and 17.6 for Kansas City, respectively. No heatstroke cases occurred in July, 1979. Heatstroke rates were 10 to 12 times higher for the elderly (ages 65 and over). Age-adjusted heatstroke ratios were approximately 3:1 for non-white versus white persons and about 6:1 for low versus high socioeconomic status. The authors suggest that prevention interventions in future heat waves should focus on the urban poor, the elderly, and minorities.

376 **Kallman, Harold. (December, 1985). Protecting your elderly patient from winter's cold.** *Geriatrics, 40*(12), 69-72, 77, 81.
    A recent study in England indicated that people prone to orthostatic hypotension are at increased risk of developing accidental hypothermia, suggesting that a history of orthostatic hypotension might be a risk factor. Because cold sensation seems to disappear after the core temperature falls below 95°F, symptoms like shivering and complaints of coldness may not exist once a patient has reached a significant level of hypothermia. As a result, hypothermia is often misdiagnosed as stroke or metabolic disorders which may exhibit similar symptoms. Bradycardia and arrhythmias are common in cases of hypothermia, as well as shallow, and in some cases almost indiscernible, breathing. Other results of hypothermia include pancreatitis and hypoglycemia. Treatment is accomplished by two methods: slow, spontaneous rewarming for most cases; and rapid, active rewarming for cases with other life-threatening complications.

377 **Kilbourne, Edwin M., Choi, Keewhan, Jones, T. Stephen, Thacker, Stephen B., Colon-Trabal, Carmen, Wassilak, Stephen G. Fite, Griffin, Marie R., Herrick, Robert F., Liang, Arthur P., Mullan, Robert J., & Patriarca, Peter A. (June 25, 1982). Risk factors for heatstroke.** *Journal of the American Medical Association, 247*(24), 3332-3336.

This case-control study assessed risk factors associated with heatstroke. The study, conducted in St. Louis and Kansas City, Missouri, took place during July and August, 1980. The authors used questionnaires to gather data for 156 subjects with heatstroke (severe heat illness with documented hyperthermia) and 462 control subjects matched by age, sex, and neighborhood of residence. Stepwise linear logistic regression identified the factors which were significantly associated with heatstroke. Alcoholism, living on the upper floors of multi-story buildings, and use of tranquilizers (phenothlazines, butyrophenones, or thloxanthenes) were all factors associated with increased risk. Factors associated with decreased risk were home air conditioning, spending more time in air-conditioned places, and living in a home well shaded by trees and shrubs. Independence, characteristic vigorous physical activity (but reducing activity during periods of increased heat), and taking extra liquids were also associated with decreased risk. Based on their findings, the authors recommend that the greatest attention during heat waves should be given to high-risk groups, and that relief efforts should include prevention and treatment measures shown to be associated with reduced risk.

378   Knochel, James P. (May, 1989). Heatstroke and related heat stress disorders. *Disease-A-Month, 35*(5), 301-377.

This journal issue is dedicated to the medical disorders related to environmental heat exposure, which are common in those working in hot climates, competitive athletes, those who exercise regularly, the elderly, and the very young. Salt and water disturbances that accompany heavy sweating in hot climates are discussed in detail, as well as the effects and implications of the resulting potassium deficiency. The major forms of environmental heat illness are heat syncope (dizziness or fainting), heat cramp, heat exhaustion, and heatstroke. These are discussed in detail with several clinical examples. Heatstroke is divided into its two major forms: classic, which affects the sedentary and confined, the elderly, and the very young; and exertional, which usually follows heavy physical work or exercise. Because severe heat exhaustion and heatstroke are life-threatening disorders, the discussion of each includes a detailed description of resulting complications and methods of treatment.

379   Lindberg, Michael C., & Oyler, Richard A. (April, 1990). Wernicke's encephalopathy. *American Family Physician, 41*(4), 1205-1209.

This article describes Wernicke's encephalopathy, a life-threatening condition caused by thiamine deficiency, that is often associated with chronic alcoholism. Symptoms may include global (total) confusion, ophthalmoplegia (paralysis of the muscles that move the eyes), nystagmus (involuntary eye movements), ataxia (disturbance of gait), hypothermia, hypotension, and other manifestations of thiamine deficiency. This condition is illustrated by the case of an elderly woman with hypothermia, confusion, and hypoxia (inadequate oxygen). After the discovery that the woman may have been an alcoholic, thiamine was given intravenously and she began to improve within a few hours. Wernicke's encephalopathy is often found in patients with Korsakoff's psychosis, a type of amnesia that occurs in alcoholics. As many as 80% of the sufferers of Wernicke's encephalopathy will also develop Korsakoff's psychosis. Alcohol withdrawal and acute intoxication can even mimic some symptoms of Wernicke's encephalopathy. Correct diagnosis of Wernicke-Korsakoff syndrome is important, because delaying thiamine treatment can be fatal. Mortality from acute cases left untreated is 17%. The condition is, however, reversible with thiamine treatment, which can be administered in large doses without causing adverse effects. The patient's response to thiamine is rapid, with improvement of eye muscle symptoms within hours, and reversal of ataxia within days of treatment.

380   **Lloyd, Evan L. (April, 1988). Hypothermia in the elderly.** *Medicine, Science and the Law, 28*(2), 107-114.

The author discusses several factors that increase the risk of hypothermia in the elderly, and suggests a number of relatively simple measures which could reduce the risk of cold-related deaths in the elderly. One source of risk is the fact that insufficient or intermittent heating is more dangerous than no heating in the house. Because hypothermia symptoms can mimic other problems like dementia or even a common cold, diagnosis is difficult. In elderly people, the symptoms are often attributed to old age rather than cold stress. Because hypothermia is often a complication of a fall or stroke, there is disagreement as to the number of actual deaths from hypothermia among the elderly. The author recommends that physicians have a high index of suspicion to discern cases of cold-related problems and hypothermia in elderly people.

381   Lloyd, Evan L. (July, 1990). Hypothesis: Temperature recommen-
       dations for elderly people: Are we wrong? *Age and Ageing, 19*(4),
       264-267.
       The author suggests that the recent reports concentrating
       recommendations to prevent hypothermia purely on housing
       temperature, particularly of the living room, may be a disservice to
       the elderly. Further, these temperature recommendations may be
       causing increased numbers of cold–related deaths, because other
       factors (malnutrition, illness, or impaired thermoregulation) can
       put an elderly person at risk of hypothermia, even when the
       environmental temperature is above the current recommendations.
       The author recommends that the elderly avoid having one room
       significantly warmer than the rest of the house, prewarm the bed
       and bedroom at night, wear adequate clothing, eat adequate food,
       and improve their level of physical fitness.

382   Macey, Susan. M. (1989). Hypothermia and energy conservation:
       A tradeoff for elderly persons? *International Journal of Aging
       and Human Development, 29*(2), 151-161.
       Hypothermia is estimated to be the sixth leading cause of
       death among elderly people in the United States. For many elderly,
       energy conservation options are often limited to little or no cost
       measures, such as turning down thermostats during winter, which
       may save energy, but which may also put the elderly person at risk
       for hypothermia. This study examined the association between the
       elderly's concern for their own health and their adoption of a
       lower winter nighttime thermostat setting. Subjects were 232
       elderly people (ages 65 and over) from Illinois and Kentucky.
       Surveys showed that the main reasons for the subjects' choice of a
       lower thermostat setting were comfort and savings. This poses a
       particular problem because of the elderly's decreased ability to
       discriminate temperature. The author recommends that other
       methods of reducing heating costs for the elderly, such as
       subsidized payments or charitable energy programs, may satisfy
       the elderly person's need to save money, while protecting them
       from the danger of accidental hypothermia.

383   Macey, Susan M., & Schneider, Dona F. (August, 1993). Deaths
       from excessive heat and excessive cold among the elderly. *The
       Gerontologist, 33*(4), 497-500.
       This study examined the demographic and other factors
       identifying those elderly people at greatest risk for mortality due
       to excessive heat or cold. The authors analyzed National Center for

Health Statistics data on elderly (ages 60 and over) excessive heat and cold deaths from 1979 to 1985. Of 5,403 temperature-related deaths during this seven-year period, 3,326 were attributed to excessive cold. Elderly males were more likely to suffer deaths from excessive cold (65.2%), and elderly females were more likely to suffer deaths from excessive heat (54.6%). Minority and rural elderly were also disproportionately likely to suffer temperature-related deaths. The authors recommend that proactive prevention programs like utility subsidies, meals on wheels, visiting nurses, home care, all of which improve general health and quality of environment, should be focused on those at greatest risk for temperature-related mortality.

384 Managing the cold weather. (December 30, 1993). *The Washington Post*, A14.

This article describes wind chill and hypothermia, and gives cold weather tips for people and pets. Wind chill is a combination of temperature and wind speed that makes the atmosphere colder than the actual temperature indicates. Hypothermia occurs when a person's body temperature drops to 95°F or lower. Symptoms of hypothermia include shivering, skin cold to the touch, rapid breathing, hyperventilation, and spontaneous urination. Cold weather tips include wearing proper clothing, staying dry, and keeping pets indoors.

385 Manning, Beth, & Stollerman, Gene H. (May 15, 1993). Hypothermia in the elderly. *Hospital Practice, 28* (5), 53-70.

Accidental hypothermia is described as a problem common in colder climates, and especially in elderly populations. Cold is not the only factor that influences hypothermia — other factors, such as disease, malnutrition, and alcohol abuse can contribute to cold stress. Because the rates of cold-related morbidity and mortality in elderly people are high, prevention is vitally important. The author recommends that physicians ask their patients about their living conditions, diet, and level of exercise, as well as drug or alcohol intake, especially in winter months when more monitoring is required due to increased risk of hypothermia.

386 Martinez, Beverly F., Annest, Joseph L., Kilbourne, Edwin M., Kirk, Marilyn L., Lui, Kung-Jong, & Smith, Suzanne M. (October 27, 1989). Geographic distribution of heat-related deaths among elderly persons. *Journal of the American Medical Association, 262*(16), 2246-2250.

This study examined the geographic relationship of elderly (ages 65 and over) excessive heat deaths by mapping data from death certificates for the years 1979 to 1985. The maps showed clusters of deaths, particularly in the central, south central, and southeast sections of the United States. The clusters were not fully explainable by population density or temperature extremes. The counties most affected were urban and, for races other than white, were relatively poor. The maps also identified counties in which heat-related health problems were particularly severe. The authors recommend that public health officials in these high-risk areas should develop heat-wave contingency plans, and that physicians practicing in such areas should be familiar with the treatment of heat-related illnesses.

387   Merchandani, H., Pace, P., Hameli, A. Z., Pressler, R., Tobin, J. G., Davis, J. H., & Melton, V. (July 23, 1993). Heat-related deaths—United States, 1993. *Morbidity and Mortality Weekly Report, 42*(28), 558–560.

Three deaths related to excessive heat exposure during hot weather may determine risk factors and prevention of hypothermia. The cases are among three different age groups: a 1-year-old infant, a 48-year-old woman and a 68-year-old man. Older people and infants are at higher risk for hyperthermia because of possible inability to get water to drink, and adults who physically exert themselves are at risk because of dehydration. Old people with illnesses are also at higher risk. Prevention measures include drinking fluids, using air conditioners and decreasing physical activity.

388   Neil, H. A. W., Dawson, J. A., & Baker, J. E. (August 16, 1986). Risk of hypothermia in elderly patients with diabetes. *British Medical Journal, 293*(6544), 416–418.

This British study examined the incidence of admissions of patients with hypothermia to determine whether hypothermia was more common in elderly patients with diabetes than in the general population. A prospective survey of three accident and emergency departments in England identified 134 cases of hypothermia admitted from a catchment population of almost 157,000 elderly people (ages 65 and over) during the winters of 1981 to 1982 and 1983 to 1984. Of the admissions for hypothermia, 23 (17%) occurred in 20 patients with previously diagnosed diabetes. Women were 87% of the diabetic admissions, and the ratio of diabetic to non-diabetic admission rates in women was 7·9. After excluding diabetic metabolic emergency admissions, the ratio was 6·4. The ratio in men was 2·4, but the small number of male admissions produced wide confidence intervals. Ten of the admissions with diabetes (43%) had other disorders that have been associated with an increased risk of hypothermia. The frequency of these conditions is higher in patients with diabetes than in the general population, and partly explains the increased risk of hypothermia in these patients.

389   Otty, Catherine J., & Roland, M. O. (August 15, 1987). Hypothermia in the elderly: Scope for prevention. *British Medical Journal, 295*(6595), 419-420.

This British study examined the effect of an educational visit from a physician on patients identified as at risk for hypothermia. Subjects were 24 patients from a register of 94 elderly (ages 75 and over) who were determined to be at risk by having two or more of the following risk factors: serious chronic diseases, history of falls or unsteadiness, malnutrition, inadequate housing, use of medications, alcohol abuse, dementia, a need to get up at night, immobility, or no regular visitors. The subjects were visited early in winter by a doctor to discuss hypothermia prevention, and subsequently revisited during very cold weather to see whether they had made any changes. Several improvements in heating arrangements were noted, but the median temperature in the bedrooms of houses with no central heating was still 10°C below the World Health Organization's recommended temperature for the elderly, young, or disabled (18°C). Despite the visits from carers and a doctor, 17 of the 24 subjects continued to live in an environment which put them at risk for hypothermia.

390   Pandolf, Kent B. (1994). Heat tolerance and aging. *Experimental Aging Research, 20*(4), 275-284.

This article is a summary of the literature on heat tolerance and aging. Work–heat tolerance has been reported to be generally lower in middle–aged and elderly men and women than in younger subjects. Other studies have suggested that physically fit older men have fewer problems with work-heat stress than do less fit men of the same age. However, none of the studies have matched older and younger individuals on any physiological or morphological variables, such as body weight, percentage of body fat, and level of exercise. Recent studies have shown that aerobic fitness and other morphological factors are important issues in the prevention of heat-related illness and death in middle–aged and elderly individuals who live and work in hot environments.

391 **Pandolf, Kent B. (Autumn, 1991). Aging and heat tolerance at rest or during work. *Experimental Aging Research, 17*(3), 189-204.**

This article reviews the literature on heat tolerance and aging. Much of the literature suggests that middle-aged (ages 45 to 64) men and women are more work-heat intolerant and suffer more physiological strain during heat acclimation, than younger individuals. It is not clear whether age differences in work-heat intolerance and physiological strain during heat acclimation are necessarily related to age. They may be associated with other factors, such as certain diseases, physical activity, and aerobic fitness. Work-heat tolerance and physiological responses during heat acclimation of active or aerobically trained middle-aged men are the same or better than younger individuals. The reviewed studies emphasize the importance of aerobic fitness and morphological factors, such as body fat, body weight, and surface area in maintaining work-heat tolerance in the elderly. Recent studies have also suggested that middle-aged and older men and women may be more susceptible to greater heat strain at physiologically significant levels of dehydration than younger people, but additional research is needed in this area. When the effects of chronic diseases in the elderly (ages 65 and over) are eliminated, levels of heat tolerance and thermoregulatory responses are comparable to younger people. In fact, healthy and well-acclimated elderly men and women appear to perform as well as younger people during exertion in dry heat.

392 **Perrone, Jeanmarie, Hoffman, Robert S., Jones, Bruce, & Hollander, Judd E. (1994). Guanabenz induced hypothermia in a poisoned elderly female. *Journal of Toxicology, 32*(4), 445-449.**

Guanabenz (Wytensin®) is a drug given for high blood pressure. There is little known about the effects of guanabenz overdose, but its structure, pharmacologic properties, and clinical course after overdose are similar to clonidine, another hypertensive drug. This article describes the case of an elderly woman with guanabenz poisoning, which was followed by hypothermia. Hypothermia has been associated with clonidine overdose, but has not been previously reported with guanabenz. The author concludes that the risk of hypothermia as a result of guanabenz poisoning is similar to that of clonidine.

393 Pinel, Carl. (May, 1989). Elderly people: Accidental hypothermia. *Nursing, 3*(37), 14-17.

The author gives a general overview of hypothermia, which is a serious but preventable threat to elderly people, especially during cold weather. Hypothermia is described as "accidental" to distinguish it from hypothermia induced for therapeutic reasons. Elderly people are at increased risk for hypothermia at milder degrees of exposure due to impaired thermoregulation, chronic illness, malnutrition, falls, and certain medications. Hypothermia can be divided into seven stages: 1. shivering; 2. confusion and disorientation; 3. amnesia; 4. cardiac arrhythmias, muscle rigidity; 5. semi-consciousness, dilated pupils, absent reflexes; 6. ventricular fibrillation; and 7. irreversible coma and death. Treatment that involves rapid rewarming is dangerous in elderly people; slow rewarming may prevent a further drop in temperature or blood pressure. The author also suggests several ways that elderly people can decrease their risk of hypothermia, such as adequate nutrition and home heating.

394 Preventing heat-induced death and illness. (July, 1994). *Health Letter, 10*(7), 1-3.

This article gives precautions to be taken for certain groups at higher risk of heat-related death or illness. The high-risk groups are infants ages one and under, adults ages 65 and over, those less able to care for themselves because of chronic mental illness or dementia, those with chronic diseases, and those who take any drug that reduces the ability to sweat or regulate temperature. The article describes the symptoms for heatstroke or collapse, heat syncope, and heat exhaustion, and gives a list of medications that may place people at risk.

395 Robbins, A. S. (January, 1989). Hypothermia and heat stroke: Protecting the elderly patient. *Geriatrics, 44*(1), 73-77, 80.

The author reviews the reasons why elderly people are more susceptible to hypothermia and heatstroke, clues for diagnosis, treatments, and practical measures to prevent the elderly from exposure to extremes of heat and cold. The elderly have increased risk because of decreased ability to regulate and recognize heat and cold, as well as a "constellation" of diseases, disorders, and other age-related factors. Because the prognosis for an elderly person with a severe heat- or cold-related illness is poor, the author suggests several methods of prevention, which include education of elderly patients about the risks and prevention of temperature-related illness. During cold weather, the elderly should be encouraged to stay indoors, to heat their homes to at least 68°F, to maintain adequate nutrition, and to wear adequate clothing. During hot weather, the elderly should avoid direct sunlight and vigorous activity, wear light clothing, use fans or air conditioners, and take adequate fluids.

396   Seipel, Michael M. O. (Fall, 1986). Hypothermia as a threat to the elderly. *Health and Social Work, 11*(4), 286-290.

The author describes the scope of hypothermia as a public health threat among elderly people. High energy costs and an increase in the number of elderly people in the United States, along with inadequate housing and other physical, medical, and social factors, have increased the numbers of elderly people at risk and suffering from hypothermia. The author recommends that social workers, along with lobbyists and other concerned agencies, actively encourage changes in public policy to subsidize heating costs for elderly people. On a local level, the author suggests that volunteer organizations and emergency units be made available to monitor the needs of at-risk elderly during cold weather. The elderly themselves should also be educated about the risks of and prevention methods for hypothermia.

397   Shuler, Thomas E., & Chillag, Shawn A. (January, 1987). The elderly and hypothermia. *Journal of the South Carolina Medical Association, 83*(1), 13-15.

This article describes the case of an 85-year-old woman suffering from hypothermia whose only apparent symptom was confusion. This illustrates how hypothermia may present itself nonspecifically in an older person. As a result, the physician may not diagnose the hypothermia because another condition will divert attention from the actual cause of symptoms. These other diseases and medical problems may also make an elderly person more prone to hypothermia. Mortality for hypothermia by itself is 10%, but when combined with other medical conditions, is 75%. The author recommends that physicians suspect hypothermia even when symptoms are not necessarily suggestive, and when temperature is not typically low.

398   Sidebottom, Janet. (August, 1992). When it's hot enough to kill. *RN, 55*(8), 30-35.

This article describes the general signs and symptoms of hyperthermia. Even though anyone may suffer a heat-related illness, the elderly, those taking certain medications, the obese, young children, people active during hot weather, and substance abusers are at increased risk. Among several types of heat-related problems, there are four major types: 1. heat syncope; 2. heat cramps; 3. heat exhaustion; and 4. heatstroke. Recognizing the signs of these heat-related problems and providing immediate treatment can help reduce the risk of complications and serious injury.

399   Simon, Harvey B. (August 12, 1993). Hyperthermia. *New England Journal of Medicine, 329*(7), 483-487.

Hyperthermia is an abnormally high body temperature that is caused by abnormalities in regulation of body temperature. Normal body temperature varies between 36.0°C and 37.5°C. It is controlled by the preoptic nucleus in the hypothalamus of the brain. This part of the brain maintains a balance between heat production and heat loss. Increased body temperature occurs when this balance is upset. There are several types of hyperthermic disorders, including exertional hyperthermia, heatstroke, malignant hyperthermia of anesthesia, neuroleptic malignant syndrome and hormonal hyperthermia. Therapeutic hyperthermia involves elevation of body temperature to treat different diseases, which has been used to treat musculoskeletal disorders and cancer. Hyperthermic disorders may cause brain damage and different types of metabolic disorders. Efforts should be made to diagnose the underlying disease in patients with hyperthermia.

400   Stout, Robert W., & Crawford, Vivienne. (July 6, 1991). Seasonal variations in fibrinogen concentrations among elderly people. *The Lancet, 338*(8758), 9-13.

This British study examined seasonal variations in physiological factors that might contribute to the increase of cardiovascular disease during winter months. Subjects were 100 elderly men and women (ages 75 and over), who were visited every month for one year. At each visit, the temperature of the home and the body temperature of the person was measured, as well as factors that might contribute to the risk of cardiovascular disease. In the course of the study, 32 subjects withdrew. Significant negative correlations were found between temperature and viscosity of the blood plasma. The viscosity was highest when the temperature was lowest. High-density lipoprotein (HDL) cholesterol, which is considered to be favorable, was also higher in the winter months. The most significant seasonal change was in the amount of the protein fibrinogen in the blood plasma. Fibrinogen, which provides the raw material for blood clots, was about 23% higher in the colder six months of the year than in the warmer months. There was no seasonal variation in blood pressure. These results may indicate that the increase in heart attacks and stroke occurring during cold weather is not related to the amount of cholesterol in the blood, but may be due to an increase in fibrinogen during this time.

401   Toulson, Stuart. (July 8-21, 1993). Treatment and prevention of hypothermia. *British Journal of Nursing*, 2(13), 662-666.

The author describes the methods of treatment and prevention of hypothermia among elderly people. Because the elderly have been shown to be at high risk for temperature-related illness, the author suggests that physicians, health care workers, and neighbors of elderly people monitor them closely, and teach them how to prevent hypothermia. The article includes several charts of symptoms, danger signs, and prevention tips.

402   Tucker, Leslie E., Stanford, James, Graves, Beverly, Swetnam, Jeff, Hamburger, Stephen, & Anwar, Azam. (January, 1985). Classical heatstroke: Clinical and laboratory assessment. *Southern Medical Journal*, 78(1), 20-25.

This study reviewed the clinical and laboratory characteristics of 34 patients with classical heatstroke during the Kansas City heat wave of 1980. The patients were elderly (mean age 67 years), predominantly black, and of low socioeconomic level. Overall mortality was 18%, with 9% of patients exhibiting severe residual neurologic deficit. Full recovery was exhibited by 73%. Patients with coma, temperature greater than or equal to 108°F (42.2°C), severe hypotension, blood coagulation problems, and need for respiratory assistance were at highest risk of death. Associated diseases were common (67%), with hypertension (32%), diabetes (21%), and alcoholism (21%) being the most common. Medications which increase risk of heatstroke were used by 56% of patients. The authors recommend that the groups at highest risk be identified during times of excessive heat, and either be provided with air conditioning, or be directed somewhere it is available.

403   Woodhouse, P., Keatinge, W. R., & Coleshaw, Susan R. K. (November 18, 1989). Factors associated with hypothermia in patients admitted to a group of inner city hospitals. *Lancet*, 2(8673), 1201-1204.

In this British case-control study that investigated random hospital admissions for hypothermia patients discovered indoors, all 14 elderly patients (mean age 80 years) studied had another serious illness. Control subjects were randomly selected from non-hypothermic admissions (ages 60 and over) at the hospital. The 14 hypothermia patients were more likely than the control group (n=28) to have been alone when taken ill (93% vs. 39%), to live alone (86% vs.43%), and to have been found on the floor (79% vs. 14%). The control group was more likely to have been wearing more than indoor clothing (50% vs. 0%), and to have heating on (89% vs. 50%), even though 93% of all subjects had heating available to them. The findings suggest that indoor hypothermia is most likely the result of a fall due to other illness when the patient is alone, lightly clothed, and not in bed. To prevent indoor hypothermia, the authors recommend using devices that enable the elderly to summon help if they become incapacitated.

10

Malnutrition

Malnutrition is not usually included in books on injury prevention, but the studies reported in this chapter attest that it is a major problem for the elderly. Malnutrition is frequently overlooked because its symptoms mirror signs of aging. Risk factors include inappropriate food intake, poverty, social isolation, disability, diseases, ethanol intake, impaired cognitive status, institutionalization, and chronic use of medication. This chapter includes articles and empirical studies on prevalence, symptoms, risk factors, special hazards, and prevention.

404 Akin, John S., Guilkey, David K., Popkin, Barry M., & Smith, Karen M. (September, 1987). Determinants of nutrient intake of the elderly. *Journal of Applied Gerontology, 6*(3), 227–258.

The authors describe a study to examine the impact of various factors on nutrient intake in a nationally representative sample of elderly people (ages 55 and over). Individual food consumption data during a three–day period were obtained for a sample of 5,615 persons from the Nationwide Food Consumption Survey. Multivariate estimation techniques assessed the effects of source of income, program participation, and demographic and personal characteristics. Federal programs, particularly those for the elderly, appear to significantly improve diet and nutrient intake. Increases in away-from-home consumption are associated with significantly smaller intakes of calcium and phosphorus.

405   Albert, Steven M. (June, 1993). Do family caregivers recognize malnutrition in the frail elderly? *Journal of the American Geriatrics Society, 41*(6), 617-622.

The author describes a case-control study to determine if family caregivers are aware of the severely underweight elder's risk of malnutrition and accordingly increase nutritional care efforts. Subjects were 125 adult daughter caregivers to frail parents. Risk of malnutrition was defined by body mass index equal or under the 5th percentile of the national average for those ages 65 to 90. The study found that, compared to caregivers of those without risk of malnutrition, caregivers of undernourished elders are significantly more likely to provide protein supplements, to make foods accessible, and to encourage and pressure the patient to eat. The author concludes that caregivers do recognize signs of severe malnutrition and subsequently increase nutritional care in response, and recommends further research on the recognition of more borderline malnutrition.

406   Arnet, Judith W., & Zahler, Lucy P. (June, 1993). Dietary intake and health habits of healthy, retired, elderly men. *Journal of Nutrition for the Elderly, 12*(3), 43-58.

Subjects were 14 retired, non-sedentary, elderly men (ages 66 to 80). The authors recorded three-day food records, one-week records of daily physical activity, and information on health habits and medical and physical activity status. The subjects' mean consumption of the selected nutrients studied were above the Recommended Dietary Allowances (RDA). The results suggest that staying active and eating an adequate diet may significantly contribute to elderly health and well-being and may delay the functional deterioration which accompanies normal aging.

407   Barrett-Connor, Elizabeth, Chang, Jae Chun, & Edelstein, Sharon L. (January 26, 1994). Coffee-associated osteoporosis offset by daily milk consumption: The Rancho Bernardo study. *Journal of the American Medical Association, 271*(4), 280-283.

This study used survey data from a southern California health study to evaluate the relationship between caffeinated coffee, milk consumption, and bone mineral density. Subjects were 980 postmenopausal women (ages 50 to 98). Eighty-eight percent of the subjects reported drinking coffee regularly at some point in their lives and 53% reported current daily coffee consumption. Smoking and alcohol use were significantly associated with lifetime coffee use. Bone mineral density of the hip and spine decreased substantially with increasing years of caffeinated coffee use. The decrease was significant and independent of age, bone mass index, cigarette and alcohol use, exercise, diuretic and estrogen use, number of live births, and years since menopause. Lifetime coffee use was only associated with bone density reductions among women who did not drink at least one glass of milk per day between ages 20 and 50.

408   Bartholomew, Anne M., Young, Eleanor A., Martin, Harry W., & Hazuda, Helen P. (December, 1990). Food frequency intakes and sociodemographic factors of elderly Mexican Americans and non-Hispanic whites. *Journal of the American Dietetic Association, 90*(12), 1693-1696.

The authors performed a dietary evaluation, using the food frequency questionnaire from the Hispanic Health and Nutrition Examination Survey, to assess the dietary patterns of 252 low-income, elderly (ages 60 to 96) Mexican Americans (n=190) and non-Hispanic whites (n=62) living in a San Antonio barrio. The relationships between food consumption and income, ethnicity, birthplace, marital status, sex, age and education were evaluated. The results of the study show that ethnicity was the important variable influencing food intake. The main difference between the two groups was in the types of foods consumed. The Mexican American diets included more poultry, meats, eggs, flour tortillas, sugar, avocados and olives. Mexican Americans also used more saturated fats in cooking, and consumed less skim milk, beef, fruits and vegetables, breads, and margarine than the non-Hispanic whites. The authors conclude that ethnicity is a major factor influencing dietary intake patterns.

409   *Be sensible about salt.* (1991). Gaithersburg, MD: National Institute on Aging.

This pamphlet discusses practical ways that older people can monitor and decrease the level of salt in their diets. Suggestions include eating foods (such as vegetables and fruit) that are naturally low in sodium, eating low-salt versions of commercially prepared food, and requesting lower sodium meals at restaurants.

410   Blanchard, James, Conrad, Kenneth A., & Harrison, Gail G. (July, 1990). Comparison of methods for estimating body composition in young and elderly women. *Journals of Gerontology, 45*(4), B119-B124.

Body composition evaluation can be helpful in determining the effect of drugs on patients, and can be important in assessing several disease states, such as severe obesity and malnutrition. Body composition refers to the measurement of fat and fat-free mass (protein, water, and bone mineral). In this study, five existing methods of measuring body composition were used to assess groups of 14 healthy young (ages 20 to 29) and 14 health elderly (ages 65 to 72) women. These methods included bioelectrical impedance analysis, regression equations involving skinfold measurements at two body sites, equations involving skinfold measurements at three body sites, body mass index, and a height and weight to total body water equation. None of the subjects had experienced any recent significant weight loss or gain, and were not on special diets for weight gain or reduction. The results indicate that the bioelectrical impedance analysis and the two methods which utilized skinfold measurements were the most effective in detecting differences in percent body fat and fat-free mass in both the elderly and the young women.

411   Brech, Detri M. (Summer, 1994). The elderly: At risk for malnutrition. *Journal of Home Economics, 86*(2), 47-49.

The author reviews risk factors for malnutrition in the elderly, and describes several methods of practical assistance that home economists and others may use to counter the risks. Current research supports the following as major risk factors for malnutrition: inappropriate food intake, poverty, social isolation, disability, diseases, and chronic use of medication. The author recommends that elderly people be taught how to make appropriate food choices, and that community programs which provide nutritious meals and social activities should be readily available. Resources available for disabled elderly, as well as information about nutrients during illness and nutrient-drug effects should also be provided and be readily available.

412   Bunker, Valda W., & Clayton, Barbara E. (November, 1989). Research review: Studies in the nutrition of elderly people with particular reference to essential trace elements. *Age and Ageing, 18*(6), 422-429.

The article describes a British study using duplicate diet analysis, metabolic balance studies and the measurement of biochemical and hematological indices to assess the trace element and overall nutritional status of 24 apparently healthy and 20 housebound elderly subjects (ages 70 to 85). Trace element status (as compared with the healthy subjects) was lower for nitrogen, zinc, copper, iron, selenium, calcium and phosphorus. The authors suggest that these nutritional deficiencies may occur more often in the elderly due to increased prevalence of predisposing factors such as living alone, depression, low income, and a housebound state.

413   Cerrato, Paul L. (September, 1990). Your elderly patient needs special attention. *RN, 53*(9), 77-80.
       The author discusses the nutritional needs of the elderly, explaining how to diagnose malnutrition and discussing some causes of nutritional disorders in old age. Routine nutritional assessment should include a complete history, a physical examination, and laboratory examination.

414   Chandra, Ranjit Kumar, Imbach, Andrée, Moore, Carl, Skelton, David, & Woolcott, Donna. (December 1, 1991). Nutrition of the elderly. *Canadian Medical Association Journal, 145*(11), 1475-1487.
       The authors review the subject of nutrition and its relevance to a growing elderly population. It is now recognized that nutrition plays an important role in health status, and that both malnutrition and overnutrition are associated with greater risk of morbidity and mortality. Certain high-risk factors may indicate nutrition problems, such as living alone, having a physical or mental disability, recently losing a spouse or friend, losing weight, using multiple medications, living in poverty, and consuming alcohol. Physical examination, anthropometry, measurements of serum albumin levels, and hemoglobin and lymphocyte counts are simple but helpful tools in confirming the presence of nutritional disorders. Prevention and treatment of nutritional problems may also prove beneficial to the treatment of common geriatric illnesses. The authors recommend a team approach in which the physician, the dietitian, and the nurse each have a defined interactive role, and that nutrition be emphasized in the training of physicians and other health professionals.

415   Coe, Rodney M., Romeis, James C., Miller, Douglas K., Wolinsky, Fredric D., & Virgo, Katherine S. (December, 1993). Nutritional risk and survival in elderly veterans: A five-year follow-up. *Journal of Community Health, 18*(6), 327-334.
       This study assessed factors which predicted survival over five years in a sample of 377 elderly (ages 55 and over) chronically

ill men. Subjects were selected at baseline from appointments at a Veterans Administration geriatric clinic and given extensive medical and psychosocial assessment. Five years later, subjects who could be located were interviewed by telephone. Interviews were completed with 194 (51.4%) subjects, 90 others were confirmed as deceased, 29 subjects could not be interviewed, and 64 more were not located, although Veterans Administration records did not show that any were deceased. The predictor variable of interest was the Nutritional Risk Index, a 16-item assessment that measures nutritional dimensions of health status. Other variables included functional health status (activities of daily living, instrumental activities of daily living), mental health status (Mini-Mental Status Exam, morale), health habits (smoking, alcohol use, and exercise), use of health services (physician visits, emergency room visits, hospital stays), and demographic factors (age, income, marital status, and living arrangements). The variables with statistically significant, direct effects on survival were younger age, higher functional health status on instrumental activities of daily living, non-smoking, moderate alcohol use, and perception of adequate income. Nutritional status was indirectly associated with survival. The authors suggest that the Nutritional Risk Index is a significant predictor of functional health status, and that it is an easily administered and effective means of screening for current nutritional health status.

416   *Constipation.* (1994). Gaithersburg, MD: National Institute on Aging.

This brochure describes constipation as a symptom rather than a disease. Constipation may be caused by medication, improper diet, misuse of laxatives or enemas, limited mobility, or physical disorders. The brochure discusses when older adults should see their doctor for constipation problems, and what, if any, home remedies may be used in minor cases.

417   Cope, Kathleen A. (March-April, 1994). Nutritional status: A basic 'vital sign'. *Home Healthcare Nurse, 12*(2), 29-34.

This article seeks to alert and inform the home healthcare nurse about the recent national focus on unacceptably high levels of malnutrition in the elderly. The author describes the significance of malnutrition in patient outcome, the Nutrition Screening Initiative's efforts to promote routine nutrition screening and intervention activities, and the simple screening tools already available to assess patient nutrition.

418 Davies, Louise, & Knutson, Kathleen Carr. (November, 1991). Warning signals for malnutrition in the elderly. *Journal of the American Dietetic Association, 91*(11), 1413-1417.

Because malnutrition in the elderly is a common but widely unreported problem, the authors review a method to assess the risk factors and warning signals of malnutrition. Risk factors are defined as identifiable biological or environmental circumstances that increase the risk of malnutrition and suggest the need for care and attention. Warning signals are observable circumstances that might then cause the at-risk patient to become malnourished. Risk factors and warning signals are usually interrelated, and the authors suggest using a grid system to evaluate this relationship for each patient. Prevention of malnutrition may only require simple first-aid techniques, such as finding a grocery store that will deliver groceries to the home-bound or encouraging proper fluid intake. Other prevention resources include community services (meals on wheels programs, social clubs), financial assistance, or, for more serious cases, medical attention.

419 Detsky, Allan S., Smalley, Philip S., & Chang, Jose. (January 5, 1994). Is this patient malnourished? *Journal of the American Medical Association, 271*(1), 54-59.

Because a variety of diseases and treatments may cause malnutrition, adequate nutritional assessment is essential. Cases cited include a 65-year-old man who became malnourished because of difficulty swallowing following a stroke, and another elderly patient who became malnourished after surgery for cancer of the stomach. A third case described is that of a 70-year-old man with a recent, unexplainable loss of 10% body weight. Despite the weight loss, and other minor symptoms usually associated with malnutrition, the patient was actually adequately nourished. The authors recommend that physicians include a detailed medical history and physical examination in a nutritional assessment, questioning patients about recent weight loss, changes in dietary habits, energy levels, and other symptoms (changes in appetite, diarrhea, nausea, vomiting), as well as evaluating loss of body fat, muscle wasting, and fluid collection.

420 *Dietary supplements: More is not always better.* (1993). Gaithersburg, MD: National Institute on Aging.

This pamphlet cautions against the overuse of nutritional supplements. Because researchers are unsure about the exact nutritional needs of older people, and because the effects of nutritional supplements are not always documented, the elderly should be particularly careful, and should ask their doctor before taking over-the-counter dietary supplements.

421   *Digestive do's and don'ts.* (1991). **Gaithersburg, MD: National Institute on Aging.**
This pamphlet gives practical advice to elderly people about a healthy digestive system. Eating a proper diet and knowing when to see the doctor are an important part of good health. The pamphlet describes common digestive disorders such as constipation, diarrhea, gastritis, heartburn, indigestion, and others.

422   **Donatelle, Edward P. (November, 1990). Constipation: Pathophysiology and treatment.** *American Family Physician,* **42(5), 1335-1342.**
This overview of constipation describes the epidemiology, physiology, evaluation, and management of this common digestive disorder. All age groups and all socioeconomic levels are affected, but the elderly are especially at risk as a result of prescription and nonprescription medications, inactivity, and disease. Other causes of constipation are congenital muscle disorders, lack of fluids and fiber in the diet (sometimes the result of bad teeth or poverty), pain, dementia, thyroid problems, neurological impairment, overuse of laxatives, and numerous other conditions. The author recommends that physicians evaluate any medications the patient is taking, including mineral supplements (even hard mineral water and antacids), antihypertensives, antidepressants, and opiates. A complete history may reveal the cause of the problem, but in some cases sigmoidoscopy, barium enema, or more specialized studies may be needed. Therapy may include behavior modification, patient education, drug therapy, and, rarely, surgery. The elderly require special care because they often have multiple and chronic problems, including malnutrition, depression, lack of appetite, poor teeth, and excessive fear of "contamination" of their bodies.

423   **Dwyer, Johanna T. (February, 1991).** *Screening older Americans' nutritional health: Current practices and future possibilities.* **Washington, DC: Nutrition Screening Initiative.**
This book discusses in great detail specific nutrition-related diseases and conditions among the elderly, as well as screening techniques and interventions. Appropriate nutritional screening should include function-related abilities involving activities of

daily living, psychosocial function and capabilities, and physical health problems. Malnutrition-related causes of disability are discussed, along with helpful interventions for older Americans. Among the areas examined are obesity, hypertension, high blood cholesterol, protein calorie malnutrition, physical inactivity and immobility, alcohol abuse, inappropriate medications, oral health problems, diabetes mellitus, renal disease, osteoporosis, iron deficiency, dehydration, constipation, chronic obstructive pulmonary disease, cancer, and other chronic degenerative diseases that require nutritional support. The book contains a comprehensive list of risk factors and screening indicators for malnutrition. The appendix contains prevalence and screening data, as well as a large bibliography.

424 Ferro-Luzzi, A., Mobarhan, S., Maiani, G., Scaccini, C., Sette, S., Nicastro, A., Ranaldi, L., Polito, A., Azzini, E., Torre, S. D., & Jama, M. A. (January, 1988). Habitual alcohol consumption and nutritional status of the elderly. *European Journal of Clinical Nutrition, 42*(1), 5-13.

This Italian study examined the relationship between habitual alcohol consumption, dietary intakes and vitamin status. Subjects were 393 elderly men (n=188) and women (n=205) ages 65 to 90 from seven retirement homes in Italy. Alcohol contributed an average of 12% of total energy intake in men, and 6% in women. Heavy drinking was identified in 48% of males and 39% of females. A general tendency for women to add alcohol to their habitual diet was shown by a positive correlation between alcohol and total energy intake. The higher energy intakes of heavy drinking women were also reflected in their higher body weights. Men tended to displace food energy partially by alcohol. Dietary risk of malnutrition did not increase with alcohol consumption. Biochemical evidence of malnutrition indicated a significant deterioration of folate status in heavy drinkers of both sexes, and for vitamin B1 in heavy drinking males only; there was no change in riboflavin status. Because plasma levels of retinol were higher and prevalence of vitamin A deficiency was lower in heavy drinkers, the authors suggest that further study should be done in this area.

425 Gallagher–Allred, Charlette R. (1993). *Implementing nutrition screening and intervention strategies.* Washington, DC: Nutrition Screening Initiative.

This manual provides step-by-step instructions for the development of programs for nutrition screening and intervention in community–based care, acute and long-term care, and outpatient or ambulatory care settings. The author describes models for the use of Nutrition Screening Initiative materials and procedures in various settings, and also highlights success stories of dietitians, physicians, nurses, dentists, social workers, pharmacists, and other health care workers. The book gives information for nutrition services professionals at local and state levels and provides practical suggestions for working with administrators and others in various health care and community settings. The author promotes interdisciplinary partnerships like the Nutrition Screening Initiative and summarizes the experiences of existing coalitions that unite the public and professionals to deliver nutrition services and health care.

426   Goodwin, James S. (November, 1989). Social, psychological and physical factors affecting the nutritional status of elderly subjects: Separating cause and effect. *American Journal of Clinical Nutrition, 50*(5 Supplement), 1201-1209.

This article reviews three factors affecting nutritional status in elderly adults: cognitive status, ethanol intake, and institutionalization. A review of the literature on cognition and nutritional status seems to indicate that subtle changes in the nutrition of older adults are partly responsible for the cognitive decline seen in elderly populations, or that the reverse is true: that cognitive decline in later years adversely affects the nutritional function of the elderly. The author's study of alcohol consumption and nutrition in the elderly appears to indicate that moderate alcohol consumption does not appear to adversely affect psychological or social status, cognition, nutritional status, or other measures of health status, a finding similar to that of younger populations. The author suggests that these results indicate that old age is not necessarily a contraindication to alcohol consumption. The nutritional status of institutionalized elderly is a complicated issue. Because malnutrition in this population is often related to chronic disease or medication, the author suggests that pharmacologists may be better suited to assess and study their nutritional status.

427   Gray-Donald, Katherine, Payette, Helene, Boutier, Veronique, & Page, Sonya. (June, 1994). Evaluation of the dietary intake of homebound elderly and the feasibility of dietary

supplementation. *Journal of the American College of Nutrition,* 13(3), 277-284.

The authors studied the dietary intake of 145 elderly subjects (ages 60 and over) receiving home care services to assess the adequacy of their intake and their ability to maintain normal body weight. In a second part of the study, they evaluated the feasibility of providing nutrient supplements to subjects at risk for malnutrition. Three 24-hour recalls, as well as height, weight and lifestyle habits were evaluated in a home interview and two follow-up telephone contacts. The effects of dietary supplementation of 14 subjects at risk of malnutrition (underweight or with substantial weight loss) over 12 weeks were also evaluated. Results indicated that mean energy intake for the entire group was low and, on average, barely matched the estimated expended resting energy. Recent weight loss was negatively correlated with energy intake among underweight subjects. Dietary supplementation resulted in an average increase in daily intake, with an average weight gain of 1.27 kilograms over the 12-week period. Weight change was directly associated with hand-grip strength and general well-being. The authors conclude that homebound elderly are at high risk of inadequate protein and energy intake, and that dietary supplementation in high-risk individuals can lead to modest weight gain and improved general well-being.

428   Greeley, Alexandra. (October, 1990). *Nutrition and the elderly.* (DHHS Publication No. FDA 91-2243)

This article describes a "nutritional twilight zone" for older Americans. The elderly tend to be at higher risk for poor nutrition, especially those in long-term-care facilities. That poor nutrition is difficult to identify, and may be diagnosed as a feature of some illness. The author explains the difficulty of encouraging the elderly to eat adequate diets and gives some practical ways to make nutritious meals more appetizing to older adults. The article includes suggestions for a daily diet and low-fat, no salt recipes.

429   Heseker, H., & Schneider, R. (February, 1994). Requirement and supply of vitamin C, E and beta-carotene for elderly men and women. *European Journal of Clinical Nutrition, 48*(2), 118-127.

The authors studied the effects of age, smoking and alcohol consumption on vitamin C, beta carotene and vitamin E requirements in elderly people. Subjects were 2,006 healthy German men and women (ages 18 to 88). Data for vitamin intake were calculated from estimated 7-day food records. The study showed that elderly non-smokers at the same level of vitamin C intake showed lower plasma vitamin C levels than younger men, an effect that was stronger in elderly smokers, indicating that elderly men may need more vitamin C in their diet to achieve comparable plasma levels. A similar, but smaller, result was shown in beta carotene levels. No age-vitamin E association was shown. The authors conclude that vitamin C, and possibly beta carotene, requirements should be higher with age.

430   Johnson, Larry E., Dooley, Pamela A., & Gleick, Jeffrey B. (September, 1993). Oral nutritional supplement use in elderly nursing home patients. *Journal of the American Geriatrics Society, 41*(9), 947-952.

The authors studied why elderly nursing home patients receive liquid oral protein supplements, what nutritional assessment the institutions used, and whether the supplements were effective. The retrospective, case control study compared 56 elderly patients (ages 65 and over) at two nursing homes who were served oral supplements at least twice daily, with a sample of 53 non-supplemented, non-tube-fed patients. Comparisons included medical diagnoses, medications, morbidity and mortality, weight changes, laboratory test results, and functional and behavioral status. The nursing home patients were given oral supplements primarily because of weight loss (71%) and poor appetite (16%). Supplemented patients were below an age-adjusted body weight on admission, unlike controls, and continued to lose weight until oral supplements were started. After beginning supplementation, the majority of case patients gained weight slowly over 9 to 10 months to approximate admission weight. Some patients on supplements showed improvement in albumin, total lymphocyte count, cholesterol, or hemoglobin, but too few patients had sufficient lab tests to verify any consistent effect. Mortality was higher in supplement patients (8 vs. 2), who were also somewhat older (87.9 vs. 84.5), but there was no statistical difference in infection or hospitalization rate. The authors also conclude that the diagnosis and prevention of malnutrition in nursing home patients is frequently disorganized, and that nutritional assessment, either for screening or for following intervention, suffers from the lack of convenient and specific assessment tools.

431 Keller, Heather H. (November, 1993). Malnutrition in institutionalized elderly: How and why? *Journal of the American Geriatrics Society, 41*(11), 1212-1218.

The author describes a Canadian cross-sectional, observational study to determine the prevalence of malnutrition and overnutrition in long-term care elderly patients and the functional, behavioral, environmental, nutritional, and medical variables associated with this prevalence. Subjects were 200 elderly patients (ages 65 and over), at a Canada long-term care hospital, who were assessed for nutritional status and the presence of specific behavioral, medical, environmental, and functional characteristics known to impact on nutritional status. Nutritional status was determined by weight, percentage of weight loss, body mass index, skinfolds, arm circumference, area measurements, and percentage of body fat. Multiple regression analyses identified the factors specifically associated with malnutrition and overnutrition in this population. Results showed that severe malnutrition was present in 18% and severe overnutrition in 10%. Mild/moderate malnutrition was present in 27.5% and mild/moderate overnutrition in 18.0%. Overnutrition was positively associated with primary diagnosis and number of medications, and negatively associated with poor appetite, number of feeding impairments, protein intake, and mental state. Malnutrition was positively associated with dysphagia, slow eating, low protein intake, poor appetite, presence of a feeding tube, and age, and negatively associated with primary diagnosis. The authors conclude that malnutrition existed at a high level (45.5%), but that this prevalence is not unusual in such an institutional setting. Behavioral, environmental, and disease-related factors greatly influence nutritional status. Malnutrition appears to be affected by nutritional factors more than overnutrition. The article recommends that prevention efforts should be directed toward influencing some of these factors to decrease malnutrition in the institutionalized elderly.

432 Kerstetter, Jane E., Holthausen, Beth A., & Fitz, Polly A. (September, 1992). Malnutrition in the institutionalized older adult. *Journal of the American Dietetic Association, 92*(9), 1109-1116.

This article examines the causes of malnutrition in institutionalized elderly in long-term and acute-care facilities. Causes include changes in nutrient requirements, medications, infections, decubitus ulcers, depression, dementia, cancer, physiologic changes that occur with age, and dehydration. Because the causes and manifestations of malnutrition in the elderly are different and more difficult to identify than in younger people, the authors suggest that standards, methods, and interpretations of nutritional assessments in the elderly should be different than those in younger adults, carefully considering the many complex physical, medical, and psychosocial factors that affect individualized nutrition care in this population.

433   **Lank, Nancy H., & Vickery, Connie E. (September, 1987). Nutrition education for the elderly: Concerns, needs, and approaches. *Journal of Applied Gerontology, 6*(3), 259-267.**

This article makes a case for the necessity of effective nutrition education programs for the elderly, a group that has a documented risk of malnutrition. The authors also describe several nutrition education programs for elderly people, including peer-educator programs at congregate meal sites, demonstrations of elderly nutritional problems and concerns at various sites, distribution of printed literature, nutrition articles in older adult-targeted publications, nutrition recipe contests, a television cooking show aimed at the elderly, public service announcements, and computer programs. These techniques have demonstrated various degrees of success, indicating those programs best suited for this population.

434   **Lansey, Stephan, Waslien, Carol, Mulvihill, Michael, & Fillit, Howard. (November, 1993). The role of anthropometry in the assessment of malnutrition in the hospitalized frail elderly. *Gerontology, 39*(6), 346-353.**

This study compared the use of percent ideal body weight and anthropometry (body measurements) in malnutrition assessment. Subjects were 47 hospitalized frail elderly patients (ages 68 to 104) at a New York geriatric hospital. Approximately 45% of patients studied had at least two anthropometric measurements below the 5th percentile, a level which indicates severe malnutrition. However, only 28% of patients were found to be less than 90% ideal body weight, a level reflecting only mild to severe changes in body weight. Serum albumin was below normal in 30% of patients. The total lymphocyte count was below normal in 53%, and was severely depressed in 24%. The anthropometry appeared more sensitive than percentage of ideal body weight as a measure of malnutrition in the hospitalized frail elderly. Because acute illness causes changes in commonly employed blood measures for malnutrition screening, anthropometry may prove to be the most stable, easily performed, and sensitive measure of malnutrition in the hospitalized frail elderly. The authors caution that further study is clearly needed, along with appropriate anthropometric reference standards for the very old.

435 Lecos, Chris W. (December, 1984-January, 1985). *Diet and the elderly.* (DHHS Publication No. FDA 85-2201)

The author describes the elderly (ages 65 and over) as the fastest growing minority in the United States, a population of men and women with unique and sometimes difficult health and nutrition problems. The elderly account for 11.1% of the total population, but represent 29% of the country's health-care costs, 25% of the prescription drugs used, 15% of all visits to doctors' offices, and 34% of all days in short-stay hospitals. The physical and even psychological changes a person experiences with aging are often influenced by lifetime lifestyle habits — diet, amount of physical activity, smoking, drinking, and medication. The chances of suffering a chronic illness are greater with age, chances that can be compounded by poor eating habits. Changing eating habits to improve nutrition can be a possible therapy for some conditions. The author gives suggestions for an adequate diet, and approaches to prevent dangerous alcohol and medication problems that can exacerbate nutritional deficiencies.

436 Lipski, Peter S., Torrance, Alan, Kelly, Peter J., & James, Oliver F. W. (July, 1993). **A study of nutritional deficits of long-stay geriatric patients.** *Age and Ageing, 22*(4), 244-255.

This British study analyzed daily dietary intakes of elderly patients with long hospital stays to determine the adequacy of their diet. The elderly patient group (n=92, ages 67 to 97) was compared to two control groups: healthy young subjects (n=41, ages 20 to 64) and healthy community-dwelling elderly (n=91, ages 71 to 93). Anthropometric (body measurement) indicators for arm values were highest for men in the young subjects group, and lowest overall for women in the elderly patient group. The relationship between anthropometric measurement and nutrition was significant for men in both control groups. The majority of elderly patient subjects had less than two-thirds of the recommended daily allowance for intake of energy (68%), vitamins D, E, and B6 (100%), folic acid (100%), magnesium (98%), zinc (98%), and retinol (90%). The authors conclude that these elderly long-stay patients were severely undernourished, and that their dietary intake (according to recommended daily allowances) did not even satisfy their basic metabolic needs.

437   **Löwik, Michiel R. H., Wedel, Michel, Kok, Frans J., Odink, Jacobus, Westenbrink, Susanne, & Meulmeester, Joanna F. (January, 1991). Nutrition and serum cholesterol levels among elderly men and women.** *Journals of Gerontology,* **46**(1), M23-M28.

This article describes a Dutch study of 539 apparently healthy elderly people (ages 65 to 79). Subjects were asked about their dietary habits, and their answers were analyzed according to the Dutch Food Composition Table. Information about their physical health, including any current use of prescriptions, was obtained through physician questionnaires. The physicians also measured the respondents' serum cholesterol levels. The results of the study indicate that there were several dietary factors significantly related to levels of serum cholesterol. In elderly men, the intake of monounsaturated fatty acids and alcohol, along with body mass index, was consistently positively associated with serum total cholesterol. The authors suggest that current guidelines for healthy diets are not age-related; in other words, that the elderly may also benefit from controlling their weight, reducing or moderating use of alcohol, and avoiding excess dietary fat.

438   *Nutrition: A lifelong concern.* **(1991). Gaithersburg, MD: National Institute on Aging.**

This pamphlet is a guide to proper nutrition for the elderly. An adequate diet should include appropriate levels of protein, carbohydrates, fats, vitamins and minerals, and fiber. These nutrients are described with a special emphasis on the nutritional needs of elderly people.

439   **Manson, Aaron, & Shea, Steven. (September, 1991). Malnutrition in elderly ambulatory medical patients.** *American Journal of Public Health,* **81**(9), 1195-1197.

The authors found that 98 of 2,986 persons ages 60 and over attending a New York hospital-based medical practice between 1979 and 1989 weighed less than 100 pounds. When their weight was compared with age-specific weight norms, all but one met criteria for malnutrition, and 62 of these subjects had comorbid conditions that could have contributed to malnutrition. The prevalence of malnutrition in this sample was 3.25%. Interviews and physical examinations of a subsample revealed that all 16 subjects either met anthropometric criteria for malnutrition, or were being treated for malnutrition. Physicians did not record a diagnosis of malnutrition or weight loss in 47.9% of subjects and did not prescribe a nutrition supplement for 76.5% of subjects. Those treated with nutrition supplements were more likely to have cancer. The findings suggest that malnutrition, both with and without comorbid disease, is relatively frequent among elderly ambulatory patients, and that nutrition is not specifically assessed or treated in many cases. The authors suggest that weight under 100 pounds in an elderly person is an accurate measure of elderly patients at risk for malnutrition.

440   Martinez, J. Alfredo, Urbistondo, M. Dolores, & Velasco, J. Javier. (August, 1990). Assessment and implications of the dietary intakes of hospitalized psychogeriatric patients. *Journal of the American Dietetic Association, 90*(8), 1111-1114.

     This study evaluated the diet and nutritional status of 390 male (mean age 58.5 years) and 384 female (mean age 62.0 years) schizophrenic patients living in a mental hospital in Spain. The food they ate during a seven-day period was recorded, and the nutrients supplied were calculated using a computer program. The patients' blood was also tested for cholesterol, iron, and hemoglobin, and patients' weight for height ratios were determined. Results indicated that women patients had low calcium intakes, and that 15% percent of the patients had reduced blood iron and hemoglobin. Zinc intakes were below the recommended dietary allowances, which is noteworthy because zinc deficiency may be linked to both schizophrenia and prolonged residence in psychiatric hospitals for the elderly. Thirty percent of the patients were overweight, even though some of them had low caloric intakes. The excess weight could be due to minimal exercise, previous weight gain, or drug therapies that can cause water retention.

441   Morley, John E., Mooradian, Arshag D., Silver, Andrew J., Heber, David, & Alfin-Slater, Roslyn B. (December 1, 1988). Nutrition in the elderly. *Annals of Internal Medicine, 109*(11), 890-904.

     The authors give a comprehensive review of the effects of anorexia and basic nutritional elements on the elderly. Anorexia is common in elderly persons, a condition often caused by unrecognized depression. Despite protein synthesis decreases in the elderly, nitrogen balance can be maintained in patients with fairly low intakes of protein. Carbohydrate intolerance is also common, but may be controlled by adequate nutrition and physical activity. Because homebound and institutionalized elderly persons often do not expose their skin to sunlight, and because the skin of older persons has a decreased ability to form vitamin D, the balance of vitamin D is precarious. Vitamins are often abused by the elderly; at the same time, certain medications may increase necessary levels of vitamin intake. Inadequate levels of zinc have been associated with deteriorating immune function, especially in those with diabetes mellitus, or in those who abuse alcohol. Zinc administration appears to protect against the deteriorating vision associated with age. Selenium deficiency seems to be associated with an increased prevalence of cancer.

442   Morley, John E. (October, 1986). Nutritional status of the elderly. *The American Journal of Medicine, 81*(3), 679-695.

The author reviews the effects and essential elements of nutrition in the elderly population. Aging affects the levels of vitamins and minerals, and the commonly resulting nutritional deficiencies can be major factors influencing some of the chronic diseases often found in elderly people. Dehydration, anorexia, protein status, lipid status, vitamins, and minerals are all discussed in detail, with a comprehensive review of current literature on each element. The elderly are particularly vulnerable to malnutrition because of normal aging, illness, decreased mobility, and economic hardship. The author makes several recommendations: 1. current educational and nutritional programs should be expanded to include women and the less educated, 2. more formal studies should be conducted in this population, 3. food technology companies should be encouraged to develop nutritionally-adequate products aimed at elderly people living alone, and 4. nutritional assessment and intervention should be promoted and subsidized as the cornerstone of preventive medicine for this population.

443   Nelson, Kristin J., Coulston, Ann M., Sucher, Kathryn P., & Tseng, Rose Y. (April, 1993). Prevalence of malnutrition in the elderly admitted to long-term care facilities. *Journal of the American Dietetic Association, 94*(4), 459-461.

This study investigated the nutritional status of elderly patients at the time of admission to a skilled nursing facility in California. Of 100 patients admitted, 39% were deemed malnourished. The results showed that patients admitted from acute-care facilities tended to be younger and more malnourished than those admitted from home. The authors suggest that the high rate of malnutrition in long-term care patients may reflect malnourished patients that were transferred from acute-care facilities. Further investigations should monitor the status of these patients in skilled nursing facilities.

444 Opper, Frederick H., & Burakoff, Robert. (February, 1994). Nutritional support of the elderly patient in an intensive care unit. *Clinics in Geriatric Medicine, 10*(1), 31-49.

The authors discuss malnutrition in the elderly, with an emphasis on the critically ill. Elderly patients are at high risk to develop protein-energy malnutrition as well as micronutrient deficiencies, a risk that increases with the onset of critical illness. An otherwise well-nourished patient can develop energy and nitrogen deficits within 7 to 10 days in an intensive care unit. The rate for malnourished elderly who become ill is much higher. Metabolic responses to injury and stress, like hyperglycemia or muscle wasting, must be understood and diagnosed in these patients. Adequate nutritional assessment includes the patient's medical history, anthropometry (body measurements), and laboratory measures of serum proteins. The authors also discuss the major components of adequate nutrients in these patients, and describe the strengths and weaknesses of different methods of nutrition delivery.

445 Rammohan, Meenakshi, Juan, David, & Jung, Donald. (December, 1989). Hypophagia among hospitalized elderly. *Journal of the American Dietetic Association, 89*(12), 1774-1779.

The authors studied hospitalized patients to determine the effects of age and gender on food intake. Subjects were 11 patients ages 65 and under and 10 patients ages 65 and over. The nutritional value of the subjects' food intake was assessed by weighing food served and uneaten. The hospital diet contained adequate amounts of energy and protein; however, 38% of the subjects ate less than 65% of their nutritional requirements. Subjects ages 65 and over showed less energy and protein intake than the younger subjects. Gender appeared to have no effect on the subjects' intake. More than 60% of the subjects (especially the elderly) had inadequate intake of micronutrients such as folate, zinc, magnesium, and vitamin B6. Multiple stepwise regression analysis showed that nutritional intake during hospital stay was predicted by the subjects' age and body weight at the time of admission. The authors suggest that the problem of hypophagia (malnutrition) in elderly hospital patients can only be prevented through more concerted efforts from doctors, dietitians, and nurses.

446   **Roe, Daphne A. (May, 1990). Geriatric nutrition.** *Clinics in Geriatric Medicine, 6*(2), 319-334.

This article is a comprehensive review of elderly nutrition, including the effects of aging on nutrition, assessment of nutritional status and requirements, current measures used to determine nutritional status, causes of malnutrition, and malnutrition-related diseases. Aging causes changes in body tissue and other physiological systems that affect the absorption of nutrients. Many other factors, such as lifestyle, mobility, medication, alcohol use, and chronic disease, also have a marked effect on elderly nutrition. The author uses several tables to illustrate suggested nutritional requirements for the elderly, risk factors for malnutrition, methods of assessment, and clinical and biochemical signs of malnutrition.

447   **Rouse, Jennifer H., & Gilster, Susan D. (1994). An improved method of documenting and evaluating nutritional intake of persons with Alzheimer's disease.** *Journal of Nutrition for the Elderly, 14*(1), 45-55.

The authors describe the many problems associated with nutritional assessment of patients with Alzheimer's disease. Because patients with dementia may forget to eat or drink in early stages, and later forget how to feed themselves or swallow, they must be closely monitored to insure proper nutrition and hydration. Recording the patient's nutrition intake is important, but often limited by the other challenges involved in feeding dementia patients. Current methods of consumption recording rely on ambiguous and non-standardized terms like "good" or "fair" which can be interpreted differently by each staff member. The authors recommend that effective documentation must be accurate, appropriate, and time-efficient. They suggest a system of standardized categories based on the percentage of foods, liquids, and supplements consumed: A (all; 100%), G (good; 75%), F (fair; 50%), P (poor; 25%), and R (refused; 0%). If the system is clear and easy for staff to use, the authors conclude that documentation will be more effective, giving an accurate picture of the patient's actual nutritional intake on a daily basis.

448 Ryan, V. Cass, & Bower, Margaret E. (December, 1989). Relationship of socioeconomic status and living arrangements to nutritional intake of the older person. *Journal of the American Dietetic Association, 89*(12), 1805-1807.

In order to examine the relationship between socioeconomic status and living arrangements to elderly nutrition, the authors surveyed 268 community-dwelling adults (ages 55 and over) in South Carolina. Of the subjects, 89% were found to have poor nutritional intake based on reported consumption of iron, vitamin B6, calcium, and vitamin A. There was no relationship between living arrangements (living alone or with others) and nutrition in this sample, but the results indicated that socioeconomic status was significantly associated with nutritional intake. The authors recommend that future studies of community-dwelling elderly should include the assessment of nutrition in high-risk groups, such as those with a lower socioeconomic status.

449 Suyama, Yasuo, & Itoh, Roichi. (June, 1992). Multivariate analysis of dietary habits in 931 elderly Japanese males: Smoking, food frequency and food preference. *Journal of Nutrition for the Elderly, 12*(2), 1-12.

The authors describe a survey of 931 elderly men (ages 65 and over) in Japan to assess the influence of smoking on patterns of diet and food preference. The results suggested that smoking decreased the taste preference and desire for fruits and vegetables. Because the Japanese get more than 80% of dietary ascorbic acid from fruits and vegetables, the authors suggest that the low levels of ascorbic acid in elderly Japanese smokers are due to a diet low in fruits and vegetables. Other studies, including several in Western societies, support this hypothesis.

450 Tucker, Katherine L., Dallal, Gerard E., & Rush, David. (December, 1992). Dietary patterns of elderly Boston-area residents defined by cluster analysis. *Journal of the American Dietetic Association, 92*(12), 1487-1491.

The authors examined the 3-day dietary records of 680 noninstitutionalized, predominantly white elderly volunteers from the Boston area (447 women and 233 men, ages 60 and over). Data were examined by cluster analysis of food contribution to energy intake. Four major high-consumption patterns were identified: alcohol; milk, cereals, and fruits; bread and poultry; and meat and potatoes. The resulting clusters differed significantly by gender, education, income, and frequency of smoking. Subjects with diets high in milk, cereals, and fruits had the highest intakes of micronutrients and the best hematologic profile. Subjects with high meat and potato intakes had the lowest intakes of most micronutrients and lowest levels of plasma folate and vitamin B6. High alcohol consumers had lowest blood levels of riboflavin and vitamin B12 and highest levels of high-density-lipoprotein cholesterol. Those with high bread and poultry intakes had lowest reported energy intakes, but had the highest mean body mass index. Total serum cholesterol and cholesterol intake did not vary significantly among groups. The authors suggest that elderly nutrition may be improved by promoting diets rich in milk, fruit, and cereals, and by counseling them to limit amounts of alcohol and meats high in saturated fats.

451   Varma, Raj N. (February, 1994). **Risk for drug-induced malnutrition is unchecked in elderly patients in nursing homes.** *Journal of the American Dietetic Association, 94*(2), 192-194.

This study assessed drug consumption patterns and corresponding risks related to nutrition. Subjects were 390 elderly nursing home patients (ages 65 and over). Data for medical diagnoses and conditions, medications taken for at least six months, weight loss from reduced food intake, laboratory tests, and nutrition supplements were taken from medical records. Results showed that frequently used drugs (such as antihypertensives, sedatives, antihistamines, laxatives, and analgesics) resulted in reduced food intake. Several of these drugs also have side effects which may include anorexia, nausea, vomiting and disinterest in food. Decreases in body weight were also noted. The author recommends several steps to prevent drug-induced malnutrition: knowing the complete drug and dietary history, understanding the potential risks associated with long-term medication use, adequately and frequently assessing the nutrition of high-risk patients, and providing the appropriate foods or supplements to prevent malnutrition problems in high-risk patients.

452   Weiner, Michael A., & Goss, Kathleen. (1983). *Nutrition against aging.* New York: Bantam Books, Inc.

This book presents a program of nutrition that will help combat most age-related disorders. It explains what vitamins and minerals to take and what foods to eat. The plan includes reducing the risks of heart disease, cancer, diabetes, and arthritis; overcoming constipation and other digestive disorders; protecting against memory problems; improving sexual virility and potency; easing the discomforts of menopause; promoting weight loss and vigor; and maintaining healthy hair and skin. The reader may score him or herself nutritionally on an ongoing quiz throughout the book. The author suggests that eating wisely and eating well will enable a person to live a longer, healthier, happier life.

453   White, Jane V. (December, 1991). Risk factors for poor nutritional status in older Americans. *American Family Physician, 44(6),* 2087-2097.

The author reviews malnutrition, an important health concern for elderly people that may result in disability, dysfunction, reduced quality of life, illness, and mortality. Inadequate food intake, chronic diseases, and disabling conditions can all increase the risk of malnutrition. Inadequate food intake may be the result of low income, inability to obtain or prepare food on a daily basis, lack of acceptable foods, lack of social support from family or friends, and living alone. Elderly patients with chronic diseases, such as anemia, cancer, mental disorders, heart disease, diabetes, high blood pressure, or thyroid disease should be screened for malnutrition. Recent history of hospitalization, surgery, trauma, infection, and involuntary weight loss should be part of any nutritional status assessment. Common medications such as aspirin, antibiotics, corticosteroids, cardiovascular drugs, antipsychotics, antacids, and laxatives can impair nutritional status. Poor oral health, tooth loss, dental caries, periodontal disease, dry mouth, denture problems, and pain can interfere with the ability to eat and contribute to poor nutrition. Factors associated with the normal aging process, such as impaired vision and hearing, can also interfere with the ability to obtain and prepare food. Loss of taste and smell can reduce the desire to eat. Because malnutrition is a preventable problem, the author suggests that regular screening and adequate intervention can help achieve the goal of a more vigorous and healthy elderly population.

11

Medication Adverse Effects and Interactions

A substantial proportion of the elderly population take one or more medications on a regular basis. These medications include prescription drugs and over-the-counter remedies. A number of problems often result which create major health problems for the patient and their caregivers. These problems include non-compliance with prescribed regimes, unexpected adverse effects, and drug interactions. The causes of these difficulties are very complex as can be seen from the materials included in this chapter. Included here are journal articles, books, and resource materials related to prevalence issues, to risk factors, specific hazards, and prevention.

454   Ali, Nagia S. (May-June, 1992). Promoting safe use of multiple medications by elderly persons. *Geriatric Nursing, 13*(3), 157-159.

This article describes guidelines for promoting safe use of multiple medications by elderly persons. The author reports that elderly people consume about 30% of all prescribed drugs and 40% of all over-the-counter medications. About 85% of the elderly residing in their own homes use medications; of these, one quarter consume an average of four drugs on a regular basis. The author describes several interventions that can reduce the chance of dangerous drug interactions.

455   Ansello, Edward F., & Lamy, Peter P. (October, 1990). *Geropharmacy and gerontology for rural community pharmacists:*

Models for dissemination. Washington, DC: AARP Andrus Foundation.

The purpose of this paper was to report the results of a project to establish partnerships with three kinds of pharmacy organizations to influence pharmacists to incorporate geropharmacy and gerontology content into their professional practices. Evaluation findings indicated that the project had resulted in significant gains in each region and that community pharmacists were engaged in complicated and challenging geriatric practices. The report also includes data regarding the prescription medication use of people ages 65 and over. In their sample, 48% were taking three to five prescription medications; 21% were taking six or more.

456   Beers, Mark H. (1992). Defining inappropriate medication use in the elderly. *Annual Review of Gerontology and Geriatrics, 12,* 29-40.

This article discusses inappropriate medication use in the elderly. Criteria for determining appropriateness is determined by examining the risk-benefit; however, for the elderly risks and benefits are not always clearly established, which leads to inappropriate prescribing. Explicit criteria generated by experts would have advantages over implicit ones. The author describes the development of applications for explicit criteria defining inappropriate medication use in the elderly using a drug utilization review concept. A set of criteria for application in nursing homes were established resulting in a list of medications that should be avoided, those whose dosage should be limited, and those whose duration should be limited. The author recommends further development of criteria for medication use by the elderly.

457   Bezon, Joan. (July-August, 1991). Approaching drug regimens with a therapeutic dose of suspicion. *Geriatric Nursing, 12*(4), 180-182.

Because of the many risks associated with giving medication to elderly people, the author recommends to approach the assessment of a patient's drug regimen with a healthy dose of suspicion. As a gerontological nursing instructor, the author developed the Individualized Drug Assessment Inventory (IDAI) to help students systematically assess polymedicine and drug doses. Nurses, however, have found the tool useful, and several now use it to help them correlate medications with individual body compositions and functions. By relating the symptoms an elderly client experiences to the side effects listed for a drug, the IDAI easily shows health care providers which elders may be suffering from the variety of medication-caused, major side effects. By highlighting side effects on the form, experienced clinicians can readily identify the offending drugs. By correlating aging body changes to how and where the drug is absorbed, distributed, metabolized, and excreted, nurses can determine if the drugs will be compatible with one another and with the aged body. One student survey indicated that the IDAI and the diagram were responsible for one nursing home's 50% drop in the amount of medications prescribed.

458   Bird, Katharine. (May-June, 1991). When advocates suspect drug restraints. *Elder Law Forum, 3*(3), 1; 5.
      This article discusses the use of psychotropics, anti-psychotic drugs, and other medications to control the behavior of elderly people in nursing homes. The author includes advice on how to check for inappropriate use of medication including checking the resident's drug history, knowing federal and state rules, and understanding drug use and the elderly.

459   Botelho, Richard J., & Dudrak, Richard II. (July, 1992). Home assessment of adherence to long-term medication in the elderly. *Journal of Family Practice, 35*(1), 61-65.
      This study attempted to quantify the extent of non-adherence to long-term medication regimens in the elderly who had one or more chronic diseases. A research assistant made home visits to 59 elderly patients. The patients' medication compliance was calculated by counting the pills. The results showed that 55% of the patients were not complying to the prescribed regime. The authors discuss possible reasons for noncompliance and interventions which might improve compliance.

460   Burns, Jennifer M. A., Sneddon, Irene, Lovell, Moreen, McLean, Ann, & Martin, Brendan J. (May, 1992). Elderly patients and their medication: A post-discharge follow-up study. *Age and Ageing, 21*(3), 178-181.
      This study assessed the medications of 56 elderly patients (ages 65 to 98) discharged from a geriatric unit who were visited at home on or after the fifth day after discharge. By the day of the visit, 15 of the 56 had not had a new prescription issued (27%) and 27 patients (48%) had old prescribed medication at home. Overall,

the medication regime started in the hospital was not being continued at home in most cases. Other problems were: inaccurately labeled containers and/or changed drug names (28%) and medications issued in childproof containers (47%). The authors concluded that poor communication between hospital and general practitioners is only part of the problem and that methods to expedite the delivery of new prescriptions should be developed.

461   Burrelle, Timothy N. (Winter, 1986). Evaluation of an interdisciplinary compliance service for elderly hypertensives. *Journal of Geriatric Drug Therapy, 1*(2), 23-52.

This study evaluated a compliance service for a group of elderly people with hypertension. Subjects were selected from 341 patients who made 9,014 consecutive visits to a medical clinic over a four-month period. Sixteen patients were referred to and participated in the Treatment Information on Medications for the Elderly (TIME) Program and these patients were randomized into control and treatment groups. Treatment consisted of home visits for psychosocial problems and instruction on compliance methods and devices. Compliance was measured by counting visits remaining in medication containers and by a questionnaire. A posttest measured knowledge on hypertension and its treatment. At the end of eight weeks, the differences in pressure reductions between the control and treatment groups were not statistically significant. Posttest scores were significantly different, averaging 96.5% for the treatment group and 73.5% for the control group. Compliance scores by unit count were also statistically different, averaging 92% and 71% for treatment and control groups, respectively.

462   Cartwright, A. (January, 1990). Medicine taking by people aged 65 or more. *British Medical Bulletin, 46*(1), 63-76.

This paper examines the relationships between aging, health, medicine consumption and consultation rates, explores evidence about medicine taking, and discusses ways to overcome deficiencies. The author found that older people consult their doctors less than younger people. Assessments of medicine taking patterns among the elderly revealed various inadequacies in supervision and a substantial proportion of questionable prescribing, such as, 4% of elderly people were taking two prescribed medicines which duplicated each other; 17% were taking medicines with potentially harmful interactions. Physicians did not know their patients and were often unaware that elderly patients lived alone, or that they drank alcohol or drove even when they were taking prescribed medicines for which drinking or driving were contraindicated. The author points out numerous other problems in the ways doctors prescribe for patients and suggests they should be audited.

463   Chrischilles, Elizabeth A., Foley, Daniel J., Wallace, Robert B., Lemke, Jon H., Semla, Todd P., Hanlon, Joseph T, Glynn, Robert J., Ostfeld, Adrian M., & Guralnik, Jack M. (1992). **Use of medications by persons 65 and over: Data from the established populations for epidemiologic studies of the elderly.** *Journals of Gerontology, 47*(5), M137-M144.

    The authors examined the extent of drug use by elders with impaired physical function, the relationship between medication use and depressive symptoms and preceding hospitalization. Samples of elderly people were drawn from four states. The subjects completed a questionnaire providing an estimate the prevalence of their prescription and over-the-counter medication use and sociodemographic and health factors related to medication use. Analysis of the data showed that 60% to 88% of the men and 68% to 78% of women used prescription drugs. Over-the-counter drugs were used by 52% to 68% of men and 64% to 76% of women. Use of prescription medications generally increased with age. Subjects reporting more depressive symptoms, impairments in physical functioning, hospitalizations, and had poorer self-perceived health status were most likely to take medications. Respondents with fair or poor self-perceived health (10% to 29%) took no prescription medications, and 3% to 13% of the sample took neither prescription nor over-the-counter medications. Use of alcohol in the preceding year ranged from 40% to 71%. The study reports medication use by age, race, education, marital status, living arrangement, income, smoking, alcohol use, physical function, self-perceived health, depressive symptoms, and hospitalizations for each of the four samples.

464   CMA Policy Summary. (1993). **Medication use and the elderly.** *Canadian Medical Association Journal, 149*(8), 1152A-1152D.

    This article presents principles for physicians to follow when prescribing medications for elderly people. General guidelines include: know the patient, consider nonpharmacologic therapy, know the drugs, keep the drug regimens simple, establish treatment goals, and encourage patients to be responsible medication users. The author outlines factors associated with physicians' prescribing patterns and includes strategies to influence those factors. Also outlined are principles that clearly define the basic steps to appropriate prescribing for elderly people.

465   Colley, Colleen A., & Lucas, Linda M. (May, 1993). Polypharmacy: The cure becomes the disease. *Journal of General Internal Medicine, 8*(5), 278-283.

This article discusses polypharmacy (the prescribing of too many medications for an individual patient) and its potential risk of adverse drug reactions and interactions. The authors describe how polypharmacy can occur and what complications ensue, they review studies evaluating interventions to reduce unnecessary prescribing, and, finally, identify practical means for the busy physician to avoid this problem. The authors recommend ways to simplify drug regimens and improve compliance such as eliminating therapeutic duplication, decreasing the dosing frequency, and reviewing the drug regimen regularly. They recommend that each patient should be on the least complex drug regimen possible and that doctors thoroughly explain the reasons why each individual is taking the prescribed medications.

466   Cooper, James H. (Fall, 1986). Drug-related problems in a geriatric long term care facility. *Journal of Geriatric Drug Therapy, 1*(1), 47-68.

This study assessed drug-related problems (DRP) in 102 long-term care patients in a 72-bed nursing home. The study was conducted over a 24-month period via a monthly drug regimen review. Assessment of patient problem list, comparison of history, established diagnoses, and drugs ordered, dispensed and administered, multimodality therapy and attainment of therapeutic/toxic end points. There were 1,224 drug-related problems (DRP) and solution recommendations in 1,728 monthly patient drug regimen reviews (0.65 DRP/review), brought to the attending physician and director of nursing attention via a consultant pharmacist monthly report. Three-fourths (930; 76%) of DRP recommendations resulted in a change of drug therapy or monitoring. Drug-related problems were placed in 14 categories with the following decreasing rank order of occurrence: medication administration and documentation errors were most common (26.5%), followed by relative drug use contraindication (16.5%), adverse drug reaction and interaction (13.1%), nutritional problem (10.5%), socioeconomic problem (10.1%), drug duplication (6.4%), drug efficacy problem (3.8%), no treatment for established diagnosis (3.8%), lab test or drug blood level need (3.4%), dosing schedule/interval change (2%), no established diagnosis but treatment ordered (1.7%), patient refusal/inability to take drug (1.5%), and drug therapy period/agent modification need (0.9%). All but one patient had a DRP with a mean of 12.0 (range 0 to 43) per patient. While this facility may not be representative of the DRP rate generally found, further studies in a large multicenter effort are needed to establish the incidence, significance, severity, cost, morbidity, and mortality characteristics of the segment of the population (i.e., geriatric age group) that displays the highest frequency of drug-related problems.

467   Cumming, Robert G., Miller, J. Philip, Kelsey, Jennifer L., Davis, Paula, Arfken, Cynthia L., Birge, Stanley J., & Peck, William A. (November, 1991). Medications and multiple falls in elderly people: The St. Louis OASIS study. *Age and Ageing, 20*(6), 455-461.

The purpose of this study was to identify associations between the use of commonly taken medications and groups of medications and the risk of falls in elderly people living in the community. A stratified random sample of 1,358 persons ages 65 and over was selected from the 15,000 members of an educational organization for functionally independent, community-dwelling elderly people in St. Louis, Missouri. Twenty-seven percent of subjects reported at least one fall in the past year and 8% reported two or more falls. After adjusting for potential confounders (including age, sex, relevant medical conditions, health status, cognitive impairment, use of alcohol, depression and use of other medications), the following medications were found to be important risk factors for multiple falls: diazepam, diltiazem, diuretics, and laxatives. The authors concluded that caution is needed before prescribing diuretics and psychotropics, especially diazepam, for elderly people. The safety of diltiazem in this age group should be assessed further.

468   Eng, Kathryn, & Emlet, Charles A. (June, 1990). SRx: A regional approach to geriatric medication education. *The Gerontologist, 30*(3), 408-411.

The issue of medication use and misuse in the older population is one of growing concern. This paper describes the Srx: Senior Medication Education Program. Eng and Emlet began by conducting a needs assessment to determine the extent of the problem in San Francisco. Surveys were sent to community pharmacists, older adults, physicians, and senior health or social organizations. Respondents confirmed the need by older patients for medication education. The program was developed and implemented in the community. By 1987, the program had reached nearly 60,000 consumers.

469   Falvo, Donna R., Holland, Beverly, Brenner, Jerry & Benshoff, John J. (May-June, 1990). Medication use practices in the ambulatory elderly. *Health Values, 14*(3), 10-16.

This study of medication use practices among the ambulatory elderly revealed a number of consistencies and inconsistencies with patterns of drug use and misuse. Medication use by the elderly is greater than use by other groups, however most studies have been conducted with older individuals with chronic or disabling diseases. Little is known about drug use patterns or problems encountered with medication use in the ambulatory, relatively healthy elderly.

470   Fincham, Jack E. & Wertheimer, Albert I. (Fall, 1986). Initial drug noncompliance in the elderly. *Journal of Geriatric Drug Therapy, 1*(1), 19-30.

This study attempted to determine whether initially drug noncompliant patients could be differentiated from initially compliant patients. The results of discriminant analysis of information provided by a questionnaire indicated that individuals in the two groups could be correctly classified at a level of 91.43%. The variables on which the initially noncompliant sample collectively scored less and which produced the most discrimination between the two groups were feedback from physicians on how to take a newly prescribed drug, belief in benefits of medical care for symptoms or illnesses, lack of physician-patient continuity, low level of satisfaction with clinic, low evaluation of self-assessed health, and inconvenience in filling new prescriptions. The initially noncompliant sample felt that physicians prescribe too many drugs, had a high opinion of self-medication activities, and did not feel prescription drugs were overly expensive. A total of 62.8% of the variance in the derived discriminant function could be accounted for by the two groups. The results pinpointed specific areas where initially noncompliant and compliant patients differ. The elderly initial noncompliant patient must be impressed with the importance of filling and taking newly written prescriptions. The lability aspects of all forms of patient noncompliance must be realized in order to impact upon the problem and to improve therapeutic interventions.

471   Fincham, Jack E. (Winter, 1986). **Over-the-counter drug use and misuse by the ambulatory elderly: A review of the literature.** *Journal of Geriatric Drug Therapy,* **1(2), 3-22.**

This review presents a comprehensive summary of impact upon seniors over-the-counter (OTC) drug taking behaviors. The authors point out that the results of OTC drug use in the elderly can be positive or negative. Positive aspects of senior self-medication can be compromised by factors that impact negatively upon the self-medication process. These factors have been shown to include the physiologic status of seniors, misinformed use of OTC drug products, misuse of OTC drugs, drug interactions with concurrently consumed prescription medications, and poorly or improperly labeled OTC packages. Because of the serious nature of potential problems, every effort should be expended by pharmacists and other practicing health care professionals in order to positively impact upon the self-medicating behaviors of seniors. Suggestions are presented for remedying the situation of misinformed use of OTC drug products which include improved patient counseling, and a heightened awareness by health professionals of potential OTC related problems in the elderly.

472   Fineman, Beverly, & DeFelice, Carol. (September-October, 1992). **A study of medication compliance.** *Home Heathcare Nurse,* **10(5), 26-29.**

This study reports results of a survey of elderly people to obtain information about their compliance behavior and knowledge of actions and side effects of their prescription medications. Subjects were 47 seniors ages 60 to 80 attending one of four senior centers in New York City. Selection was restricted to people who were taking one or more medications, ages 60 and over, functioning independently, able to administer their own medications, and willing to sign informed consent. Results indicate a need for health care professionals to continue to assess client medication knowledge and identify variables that interfere with recall and retention of previous learning.

473   Finlayson, Richard E. (1984). **Prescription drug abuse in older persons. In Roland M. Atkinson (Ed.),** *Alcohol and drug abuse in old age* **(pp. 61-69). Washington, DC: American Psychiatric Press, Inc.**

The purpose of the study was to study prescription drug abuse among the elderly. Finlayson examined the histories of 248 people ages 65 and over treated at an alcohol and drug dependency unit. Of these, 214 (86%) were dependent on alcohol alone; 19 (8%) were dependent on prescription drugs alone; and 15 (6%) were dependent on a combination of prescription drugs and alcohol. Types of drugs abused were analgesics, alcohol, tranquilizers, and sedative/hypnotics. Reasons given for most recent drug use were pain (53%), insomnia (21%), marital/family discord (21%), retirement/death of spouse (15%), work stress (12%), and depression (9%). Finlayson identifies several conditions in the elderly that should alert clinicians to a possible drug abuse problem — pain disorders, depression, organic mental disorders, low levels of psychosocial functioning, change in tolerance to drugs, accident proneness, and defensiveness. He recommends physician education of patients as the most useful method of primary prevention.

474   Gehres, Robert W. (Winter, 1986). **A medication monitoring service for elderly patients offered by the pharmacist on a fee-for-service basis.** *Journal of Geriatric Drug Therapy, 1*(2), 81-90.

This paper describes a medication monitoring service (MMS) for elderly residents of a congregate housing facility provided by the pharmacist on a fee-for-service basis. The MMS entails repackaging prescribed medications into customized medication packaging (seven-day supply) and weekly home visits by the pharmacist. During these visitations the pharmacist 1. monitors for medication compliance, 2. counsels that patient regarding his/her drug therapy, 3. monitors for drug efficacy and drug toxicity, and 4. provides verbal reinforcement to enhance compliance and retention of information. In addition, the pharmacist consults with the patient's physician and responsible family member concerning drug therapy problems or a change in health status. The MMS was evaluated for its effect on medication compliance. The mean compliance for a subgroup of eight patients over a six-month period was 92% and ranged from 73% to 100%. In addition, the MMS was evaluated for its effect on physician prescribing. During a period of two years a total of 42 changes in drug therapy were made for this subgroup. Of these changes, 17 were the direct result of intervention by the pharmacist. Interventions were usually prompted by the development of adverse drug reactions or therapeutic failure. The MMS has been a useful home care pharmacy service for geriatric patients whose primary limitation to independent living is medication compliance.

475 **Gerety, Meghan B., Cornell, John E., Plichta, Denise T., & Eimer, Michelle. (1993). Adverse effects related to drugs and drug withdrawal in nursing home residents.** *Journal of the American Geriatrics Society, 41,* 1326-1332.

The purpose of the study was to develop and standardize explicit criteria to link clinical adverse events to drug withdrawal, determine the incidence and severity of Adverse Drug Events (ADE) and Adverse Drug Withdrawal Events (ADWE) in a nursing home population, and establish the contribution of demographic, clinical, and functional characteristics to ADE and ADWE. Subjects were mostly (96%) men, ages 70 and over, and taking an average of seven medications. Results indicated that 95 residents experienced 201 ADE. Of the sample, 12 required hospitalization and one resident died. Also, 62 patients had 84 ADWE. One was associated with hospitalization, and none were associated with death. The most common risk factors were number of diagnoses, number of medications, and hospitalization during the nursing home stay. The authors concluded that ADE and ADWE were common in nursing home residents in this Veterans Affairs setting. Explicit criteria developed and applied in this setting should be applied prospectively in other settings to further define risk of drug discontinuation and to assist in development of specific drug discontinuation guidelines.

476 **Gillin, J. Christian, & Byerley, William F. (January 25, 1990). Drug therapy: The diagnosis and management of insomnia.** *New England Journal of Medicine, 322*(4), 239-248.

This comprehensive review article discusses insomnia, its causes and variability. The authors recommend assessing the patient's life events, medications, psychological and medical factors upon diagnosis. Causes of short-term insomnia and chronic insomnia vary and the problem should reflect those differences. Treatment should be directed at the underlying causes, and may involve withdrawal of substances causing side effects, management of stress, counseling, and various psychotherapeutic techniques. Sleeping pills may be used for transient, short-term insomnia, but are not recommended for long-term treatment. Benzodiazepines are the drugs of choice for insomnia, and consist of various long-and short-acting forms. Long-acting drugs such as flurazepam produce sedative hangover effects the next day, whereas short-acting agents such as triazolam may worsen the insomnia and cause a form of amnesia. Because side effects are related to dose, the dose should be kept low. When prescribing hypnotics, a physician should take into consideration the patient's age and lifestyle and duration of treatment, and avoid large or renewable prescriptions. Depressed or suicidal patients, alcohol or substance abusers, the elderly and mentally impaired, patients with sleep-related breathing disorders and incurable insomnia, and pregnant women require special attention.

477   Green, Lawrence W., Mullen, Patricia D., & Stainbrook, Gene L. (Fall, 1986). Programs to reduce drug errors in the elderly: Direct and indirect evidence from patient education. *Journal of Geriatric Drug Therapy, 1*(1), 3-18.

This review examined ten experimental studies specifically addressing the elderly with educational and behavioral interventions designed to improve their compliance. Except for program using written materials used alone, each program resulted in significantly and substantially improving the subjects' knowledge, drug errors and/or clinical effects. In one study specifically comparing the effects of a patient education program on older and younger hypertensive patients, the old patients showed significantly greater gains in compliance, appointment-keeping, and blood pressure control. The authors conclude that the elderly are sufficiently motivated to overcome the major disadvantages and deficits they face in managing their medical regimens. Programs to support their motivations should concentrate on enabling factors such as the physical and monetary attributes of the drug regimen. The old-old (ages 75 and over) require particular attention to these aspects of prescribed medications.

478   Hahn, Karen, & Wietor, Gail. (May-June, 1992). Helpful tools for medication screenings. *Geriatric Nursing, 13*(4), 160-166.

This article describes the development, testing, and revision of a medication screening tool to assist with identifying some of the complex problems related to medication use by elderly patients. Subjects of the try-out were clients at a monthly blood pressure screening at a federally subsidized apartment building. Of the 20 clients, 18 reported taking medications; three (16%) of these 18 had potentially life-threatening noncompliance problems.

479   Hanlon, Joseph T., Fillenbaum, Gerda G., Burchett, Bruce, Wall, William E., Jr., Service, Connie, Blazer, Dan G., & George, Linda K. (1992). Drug-use patterns among black and nonblack community-dwelling elderly. *The Annals of Pharmacotherapy, 26*(5), 679-685.

The purpose of the study was to describe and compare drug-use patterns among black and nonblack community dwelling elderly. The study sample was 4,164 community residents ages 65 and over (mean age 73.56 years) from the Piedmont Health Survey of the Elderly, which is part of a study funded by the National Institute on Aging. The data were collected through an in-home interview. The sample included 54% blacks; 44.6% whites; and 1.6% Hispanics, American Indians, and Asians. Overall, 75% used one or more prescription drugs; 72% used one or more over-the-counter drugs, 91% used either one prescription or one over-the-counter drugs. Blacks differed little from nonblacks in use of prescription drugs; they were less likely to be using over-the-counter drugs.

480   Jenner, Gillian. (1993). Prescribing in the elderly. *The Practitioner, 237*, 450-452.

This article presents information regarding prescribing medications for elderly people including physiology and drug handling, principles of prescribing, some commonly used drugs, and rules of prescribing. Information about different absorption and distribution rates that affect medication effects is explained. Drugs discussed are: diuretics, digoxin, antihypertensives, night sedation, antidepressants, opiate analgesics, antiepileptics, antiparkinsonian drugs, and non-steroidal anti-inflammatory drugs. The author lists cardiovascular drugs and central nervous system drugs and other drugs commonly causing adverse reactions in the elderly and includes a list of those adverse reactions. He says that drug therapy can be of great help to the elderly, when used wisely and recommends that emphasis be on simple regimes and proper supervision to avoid over-treatment and drug interactions, and producing benefit while avoiding major adverse reactions.

481   Juergens, John P., Smith, Mickey C., & Sharpe, Thomas R. (Fall, 1986). Determinants of OTC drug use in elderly. *Journal of Geriatric Drug Therapy, 1*(1), 31-46.

This study examined the determinants of over-the-counter (OTC) drug use in an elderly population. The sample consisted of

300 persons ages 60 and over residing in Tupelo, Mississippi and the surrounding county. Data were collected using household interviews. Questions pertained to demographic characteristics, transportation, availability and access to medical and pharmaceutical services, perceptions of health, and the use of prescribed and non-prescribed (OTC) drugs. Drug use was defined as the number of medicinal products reported consumed in a two-week period before the interview. Identification of the determinants of heavy OTC drug use was accomplished through multiple discriminant analysis. A combination of demographic, availability and access, and psychosocial variables was most important in developing a profile of heavy OTC drug users in this population. This study found black males living in rural areas to be the heaviest users. Higher OTC drug use was associated with lower income and education.

482   Kofoed, Lial L. (1984). Abuse and misuse of over-the-counter drugs by the elderly. In Roland M. Atkinson (Ed.), *Alcohol and drug abuse in old age* (pp. 50-59). Washington, DC: American Psychiatric Press, Inc.

This chapter discusses problems with the use of over-the-counter drugs by the elderly. The author discusses reasons why elderly people use more OTC drugs than other groups, the special risks of OTC drug use by older people, and major OTC drug groups (analgesics, laxatives, antihistamines and anticholinergics, sympathomimetics, alcohol containing compounds, and others). He also includes caffeine and nicotine in his discussion of OTC drugs. Kofoed states that treatment is difficult to discuss because misuse is more common than abuse. He calls for physician and patient education to prevent adverse reactions and drug interactions. He concludes that older people are very likely to use OTC drugs and are at increased risk for adverse reactions, drug interactions, and side effects.

483   Kofoed, Lial L. (October, 1985). OTC drug overuse in the elderly: What to watch for. *Geriatrics, 40*(10), 55-60.

This article describes the use patterns, side effects, and drug interactions of the various OTC drug categories and can help the primary care physician diagnose OTC drug misuse or abuse in the elderly patients. Older people with limited mobility or incomes may choose OTC drugs for self-treatment rather than visit a physician especially for treating arthritis, insomnia, or constipation. The author describes diagnostic clues to recognize misuse or abuse of analgesics, laxatives, antihistamines and anticholinergics, sympathomimetics, alcohol-based drugs, caffeine, and nicotine. The author recommends early diagnosis as the key to stopping OTC misuse or abuse and prevention through patient education.

484   Langan, Michael L. (March-April, 1993). A prescription drug monitoring system to record drug histories, reduce 'misadventures'. *Public Health Reports, 108*(2), 173-174.

This article describes a system for monitoring prescription drug use among elderly people. The PHARMACARD system includes a credit card-type optical card to store prescription histories and information, an optical card reader with a computer at the pharmacy, and a computer program to maintain records and databases. The software would record the person's personal and medical history, a prescription history, and a database of drug interactions. The PHARMACARD system will be tested with 200 volunteers and their local pharmacies.

485   LeSage, Joan. (June, 1991). Polypharmacy in geriatric patients. *Nursing Clinics of North America, 26*(2), 273-289.

This review discusses the scope of polypharmacy, settings, causes, problems and health risks, and prevention. While the practice of multiple drug prescriptions is denounced in geriatric literature, it is common in nursing homes and occurs less often among the community-dwelling elderly. Possibly it is related to the higher incidence of chronic disease in older adults rather than chronological age. Available data suggest possible causes, health risks, and areas for intervention. Polypharmacy can be associated with increased adverse drug reactions, drug interactions, and medication errors. Prevention should include comprehensive baseline assessment and periodic reassessment to determine need for and efficacy of prescribed drugs, attempts at nondrug therapy, improved provider drug prescription and administration practices, and promotion of safe self-medication behavior. Health risks associated with polypharmacy and the escalating cost of medications require that nurses participate in efforts to ensure that the elderly receive only necessary and effective drug treatment.

486   Lindley, C. M., Tully, M. P., Paramsothy, V., & Tallis, R. C. (July, 1992). Inappropriate medication is a major cause of adverse drug reactions in elderly patients. *Age and Ageing, 21*(4), 294-300.

The authors investigated the extent to which adverse drug reactions (ADR) in elderly patients admitted to hospital are due to inappropriate prescribing. Subjects were 416 successive admissions of elderly patients to a teaching hospital. Interacting drug combinations and drugs with relative contra-indications (CI) were common, but not as important in producing ADR as drugs with absolute CI or unnecessary drugs. Forty-eight patients (11.5% of admissions) were taking a total of 51 drugs with absolute CI (3.8% of prescriptions). One hundred and seventy-five drugs were discontinued on or shortly after admission in 113 (27%) patients because they were deemed to be unnecessary. One hundred and three patients (27.0% of those on medication) experienced 151 ADR, of which 75 (49.7%) were due to drugs with absolute CI and/or that were unnecessary. A significantly higher rate of ADR, 13 (50%), were due to inappropriate prescriptions. The admission rate per prescription was significantly higher ($p < .001$) for inappropriate than for appropriate drugs. The authors concluded that much drug-related morbidity in the elderly population is due to inappropriate prescribing and may be avoidable.

487   Livingston, Jenny, & Reeves, Robert D. (October, 1993). Undocumented potential drug interactions found in medical records of elderly patients in a long-term-care facility. *Journal of the American Dietetic Association, 93*(10), 1168-1170.

This article describes a study to determine potential drug interactions among elderly nursing facility residents. The authors examined medical records of 52 residents (9 men, 43 women) in an intermediate-care facility. Their prescriptions were recorded and evaluated according to drug, frequency, and time of administration with regard to meals. The medical records contained no written record of potential drug or drug-nutrient reactions, but only 13 of the subjects were actually free from such reactions. The authors describe age- and pharmacokinetic-related factors that affect adverse drug reactions in the elderly, and recommend that health care professionals be aware of such reactions via the patient's medical record.

488   Maloney, Susan K., & Ury, Wayne A. (1987-1988). Using medicines safely—for a better life: Findings from the healthy older people program. *Journal of Geriatric Drug Therapy, 2*(2/3), 127-138.

This article discusses the findings from the Healthy Older People Program, a nationwide health promotion program which has been implemented with two sets of desired outcomes: 1. to educate older adults about behaviors to improve health, including appropriate medication use; and 2. to stimulate the development or expansion of community-based programs. The program has three major components: developing consumer materials, establishing a nationwide distribution network, and establishing training and technical assistance. The program has drawn on already existing research in putting together and disseminating public education materials. A program such as Healthy Older People can have a significant impact upon the knowledge and behavior of the growing number of older adults in the United States who use prescription and over-the-counter drugs and can stimulate professionals in the health and aging fields to be more aware of medication issues.

489   McKenzie, Lynda C., Kimberlin, Carole L., Pendergast, Jane F., & Berardo, Donna H. (1994). **Potential drug interactions in a high risk ambulatory elderly population.** *Journal of Geriatric Drug Therapy, 8*(3), 49-63.

This study investigated the rates of occurrence of potential drug–drug interactions in ambulatory patients ages 60 and over taking medications to treat chronic conditions and examined the variables which differentiated patients with potential drug–drug interactions from patients who had no interactions. Volunteer community pharmacists (N=102) enrolled 762 patients who met criteria on use of medications for chronic conditions into the study. Detailed medication histories were obtained for these patients through telephone interviews. Eighty-two patients (10.8%) had at least one potential drug interaction. Ninety-five percent of patients with at least one drug–drug interaction were taking four or more prescription drugs concurrently. The number of prescription drugs taken by patients with at least one potential drug interaction (mean=8.1, SD=3.1) was significantly higher (t=3.48, p < .001) than the number being taken by those with no interactions (mean=6.2, SD=2.9). For each additional medication, the probability of having at least one drug interaction increased by 22.4% (controlling for age of the patient, having more than one prescribing physician and obtaining prescriptions from more than one pharmacy). None of the other variables in the model were significantly related to the probability of having an interaction. The drugs most commonly involved in the drug interactions were potassium sparing diuretics and potassium replacement products. Nine other drug interactions are listed. Side effects of interactions listed in the article include dyspepsia, insomnia, rectal bleeding, indigestion, rash, and others. The primary finding is that the risk of problems is associated with the number of drugs taken.

490   McMurdo, Marion E. T., Jarvis, Andrew, Fraser, Callum G., & Ghosh, Uptal K. (1991). A novel approach to the assessment of drug compliance in the elderly. *Gerontology, 37,* 339-344.
        This pilot study examined the use of a qualitative thin-layer chromatographic technique (Toxi-Lab system) applied to urine specimens in assessing drug compliance in the elderly. The system proved capable of detecting 36% of prescribed drugs in a group of elderly patients, and offers a different and inexpensive approach to monitoring compliance with certain medications.

491   *Medication management in homes for adults and non-medical rehabilitation centers.* [videotape] (1993). Richmond, VA: Virginia Department of Social Services.
        This 53-minute video and questionnaire presents information about medication management in homes for adults and non-medical rehabilitation centers. Medication management in homes for adults or non-medical rehabilitation centers was designed to supplement *A Resource Guide for Medication Management for Agents Authorized under the Drug Control Act* prepared for programs licensed by the Virginia Departments of Social Services, Mental Health, and Mental Retardation Trainers can use this video with individual trainees or classes. For train-the-trainer sessions, the video can be used to illustrate the presentation of a lesson covering several tasks.

492   Messner, Roberta L., & Gardner, Sylvia S. (January, 1993). Start with the medicine cabinet. *RN, 56*(1), 50-53.
        This article provides ideas on how to perform a detailed evaluation of a patient's medication history. This procedure is a necessary to prevent inappropriate drug usage that usually results in adverse side effects. The elderly face the greatest risk, and therefore, require special attention. Inquiring about past and present prescription or over-the-counter medications, giving information on medication expiration, proper storage of various drugs and learning about a patient's eating habits and lifestyle are recommended ways to effectively assess a patient's medical history.

493 Murray, Michael D., Birt, Julie A., Manatunga, Amita K., &
Darnell, Jeffrey C. (May, 1993). **Medication compliance in elderly
outpatients using twice-daily dosing and unit-of-use packaging.**
The Annals of Pharmacotherapy, 27(5), 616-621.

This study investigated the effect of unit-of-use drug
packaging of medications on compliance among elderly
outpatients treated with complex medication regimens. The
settings were geriatric outreach health centers in urban public
housing units for independent-living elderly people. Subjects were
31 adults ages 60 and over, each taking three or more prescribed
medications, who were randomly assigned to one of three study
groups: group one (n=12), no change in dosing or packaging;
group two (n=10), conventional packaging with twice-daily
dosing; group three (n=9), unit-of-use packaging with twice-daily
dosing. The intervention was a unit-of-use package consisting of a
two-ounce plastic cup with a snap-on lid containing all
medications to be taken at the time of dosing. The main outcome
measures for medication compliance was assessed monthly for six
months using tablet counts. Medication compliance was
significantly better in group three (92.6%) using unit-of-use
packaging compared with either group one (79%) or group two
(82.6%). Compliance did not differ between groups 1 and 2. In this
small study of elderly outpatients taking three or more
medications, unit-of-use packaging and twice-daily dosing
improved medication compliance compared with conventional
packaging.

494 Nathan, David M. (November, 1990). **Insulin treatment in the
elderly diabetic patient.** *Clinics in Geriatric Medicine,* 6(4), 923-
929.

This article discusses the use of insulin treatment in Type II
diabetic mellitus patients, who comprise approximately 20% of the
United States elderly population. Since there is no empirical
evidence that supports the need to maintain a specific level of
glucose beyond that necessary to relieve symptoms, the choice of
therapy is problematic. Clearly, supervised dietary therapy for the
obese Type II diabetic patient represents a safe and cost-effective
treatment. For those patients who fail dietary therapy because they
fail to lose weight of regain lost weight, or because blood glucose
levels remain high despite weight loss, further therapy must be
individualized. In the author's view, the best criteria for drug
treatment are 1. persistent symptoms associated with
hyperglycemia, 2. ketonuria in the unstressed state, and 3. certain

cases of hyperlipidemia, especially with high triglyceride levels. In these situations, drug therapy is necessary to eliminate symptoms, prevent development of ketoacidosis, and reduce the risk of pancreatitis, respectively. Physicians should also consider drug therapy in the case of very elevated blood glucose levels, even in the absence of symptoms, when dehydration and risk of severe hypersmolarity exist.

495   National Institute on Aging. (1991). Safe use of medications by older people. *Age Page*, 1-2.

This paper discusses the effectiveness and availability of drugs, vaccines, and medicine and warns that over-the-counter drugs, while useful, may contain strong agents that can have dangerous side effects. A list of suggestions that can reduce the risk of medication use is included.

496   Ory, Marcia G. (1987/1988). Social and behavioral aspects of drug-taking regimens among older persons. *Journal of Geriatric Drug Therapy*, 2(2/3), 103-114.

The purpose of this paper is to 1. discuss, in general terms, the linkage between health and behavior; 2. review how aging processes influence the interrelationships between health and behavior; 3. highlight the dynamic processes involved in the continuum of illness behaviors from symptom recognition to compliance to prescribed regimens; 4. report biological, behavioral, and social influences on drug-prescribing and drug-taking behaviors for older persons; and 5. recommend future research directions. Older people on average have more chronic diseases and disabilities than younger persons are therefore more likely to use more medications both prescription and over-the-counter. Ory discusses reasons for noncompliance with prescribed drug regimes and remarks that it is one of the most difficult problems encountered by physicians. The author describes several areas where research is needed including: information about the relationship between health, drug-taking behaviors and lifestyle factors such as exercise and nutrition, the stability of drug compliance behaviors over the life course, influences of age, gender and ethnicity on symptom recognition and health seeking behaviors, identifications of older people at high risk for compliance problems or adverse drug side effects, algorithms for distinguishing illness symptoms from drug side effects in older people, and others.

497   Ouslander, Joseph, Schnelle, John, Simmons, Sandra, Bates-Jensen, Barbara, & Zeitlin, Michael. (April, 1993). The dark side of incontinence: Nighttime incontinence in nursing home residents. *Journal of the American Geriatrics Society, 41*(4), 371-376.

This prospective study describes the characteristics of nighttime urinary incontinence in a sample of nursing home residents in four settings. Subjects were 136 incontinent nursing home residents. The measurements were frequency and volume of incontinent and continent voids for three 10-hour daytime and three 10-hour nighttime data collection periods. It resulted in the frequency of nighttime incontinence was the same as during the day, but the volume of nighttime incontinent voids and total nighttime volume were higher than during the day. There was substantial between-and within- subject variability in volumes, but the distribution of ratios of night/total volumes approximated a normal curve. Diuretic use was associated with relatively low nighttime volumes. The researchers concluded that about one-quarter of the nursing home residents produced substantially more urine at night than during the day. They recommended consideration of several medical, behavioral, and environmental approaches for reducing the frequency and volume of nighttime incontinence in this population.

498   Petersen, David M., Whittington, Frank J., & Payne, Barbara P. (Eds.). (1978). *Drugs and the elderly: Social and pharmacological issues.* Springfield, IL: Charles C. Thomas.

This book provides a practical guide on drugs and the elderly. The first part includes several chapters which describe the problem and define the issues. A summary of major research findings related to use and misuse of alcohol and drugs is also provided. The second part of the book provides information about pharmacology and pharmacy as they related to the elderly including drug side effects, drug interactions, and the problems of self-medication, and the role of pharmacies. The final section addresses clinical and community responses to elderly drug use primarily by physicians, nurses, and other care providers.

499   Poff, Gregory A., Mutnick, Alan H., & Swanson, Larry N. (Winter, 1986). An assessment of pharmacist intervention in a geriatric day care center setting. *Journal of Geriatric Drug Therapy, 1*(2), 53-66.

This study investigated the impact of a clinical pharmacist in two of geriatric day care centers in the Boston area. A clinical pharmacist provided a defined set of services which focused on drug therapy monitoring. Drug therapy recommendations were mailed to the physicians responsible for the care of the clients at these settings. An independent panel consisting of two clinical pharmacists and a physician rated these recommendations as "definitely" or "probably" significant in almost two-thirds (61.3%) of the cases. For those physicians responding, over half (54.5%) of the pharmacist's suggestions were accepted. The total number of medications and the frequency of drug administration were decreased by the pharmacist. It was concluded that these patients do not have extensive medication problems but several significant drug therapy changes were made. The author concluded that this area of pharmacist involvement warrants further study.

500   Pollow, Rachel L., Stoller, Eleanor Palo, Forster, Lorna Earl, & Duniho, Tamara Sutin. (January-February, 1994). Drug combinations and potential for risk of adverse drug reaction among community-dwelling elderly. *Nursing Research, 43*(1), 44-49.

This study investigated drug combinations and potential adverse drug reaction risk. Data were gathered through personal interviews from a sample of 667 people ages 65 and over living independently in community settings Almost two thirds of these older respondents reported at least one drug-drug or drug-alcohol combination associated with a possible adverse reaction. The largest percentage of respondents were taking combinations of medications that could place them at risk for hypotension and cognitive impairment. The author concluded that more detailed screening of specific medications used by older people who report taking certain categories of drugs was needed.

501   Ried, L. Douglas, Christensen, Dale B., & Stergachis, Andy. (1990). Medical and psychosocial factors predictive of psychotropic drug use in elderly patients. *American Journal of Public Health, 80*(11), 1349-1357.

This study investigated medical and psychosocial factors that may be used to identify patients at risk of psychotropic drug use. Population-based surveys were completed by 278 elderly health maintenance organization (HMO) patients in August, 1984. Physical and mental health status and social support were measured in the survey. Automated prescription records from the year prior to and the year after the survey were linked to data from the survey. Patients received 737 prescriptions for psychotropic drugs during the two-year period under study. Doxepin (20.2%), flurazepam (15.2%), and diazepam (14.8%) were dispensed most frequently. Nearly 30% of the patients received a prescription for at least one psychotropic drug during the two-year period, and 14% received at least one prescription during both years. Three significant predictors of subsequent psychotropic drug use were: prior use, the number of physical impairments, and the respondents' rating on the Alameda Health Scale. Patients' self-reported mental health status and sociodemographic characteristics were not significant predictors of subsequent use.

502   **Rodman, Morton J. (January, 1993). OTC analgesics and anti-inflammatories.** *RN, 56*(1), 54-60.

This article lists the three most common over-the-counter analgesics and anti-inflammatories and medications and substances that may interact with them. They are acetaminophen (Tylenol), aspirin, and ibuprofen (Advil, Motrin). The author reports that therapeutic doses of acetaminophen with alcohol can cause liver damage in chronic alcohol abusers. Interactions may also occur when taken with oral anticoagulants, certain anti-seizure drugs, sulfinpryrazone, charcoal, and food. Aspirin can be dangerous if combined with oral anticoagulants, heparin, thrombolytic agents, alcohol, antacids, and other medications. Among the medications that can interact with ibuprofen or reduce its effectiveness are heparin, diuretics, aspirin, and food.

503   **Rousseau, Paul, & Fuentevilla-Clifton, Ana. (August, 1993). Acetazolamide and salicylate interaction in the elderly: A case report.** *Journal of the American Geriatrics Society, 41*(8), 868-869.

This case report illustrates an adverse interaction between acetazolamide and salicylate. The author points out that glaucoma and arthritis are common chronic disorders among the elderly, often necessitating pharmacologic intervention for appropriate management. Acetazolamide and salicylates are commonly prescribed in glaucomatous and arthritic elders, predisposing them to a deleterious drug-drug interaction with elevated serum levels of acetazolamide and a clinical syndrome consisting of fatigue, lethargy, somnolence, incontinence, and confusion. He warns that clinicians are often unaware of this drug-induced syndrome and persist in the concurrent use of acetazolamide and salicylates.

504   Salzman, Carl. (February, 1991). The APA Task Force Report on benzodiazepine dependence, toxicity and abuse. *American Journal of Psychiatry, 148*(2), 151-152.

This editorial is a discussion of the results of the American Psychiatric Association Task Force Report on benzodiazepine dependence, toxicity, and abuse. Benzodiazepines are central nervous system depressants commonly prescribed for the short-term treatment of anxiety, stress or insomnia. The APA task force found that although therapeutic use is usually limited to 60 days or less, a substantial number of adults (1.65% of the population) have been taking benzodiazepines for one or more years. Short-term treatment with standard therapeutic doses rarely proves harmful. However, high doses or prolonged periods of use can result in toxicity or dependence, particularly among people who also abuse alcohol, opiates, cocaine or other sedatives. Dependence is also more likely to occur among individuals with a past history of alcoholism. The author points out that elderly patients are particularly sensitive to benzodiazepine toxicity, which can lead to confusion, unsteadiness and falling down. Withdrawal symptoms, which can include seizures and psychotic episodes, usually occur only after prolonged treatment with high doses. It is important to slowly taper off these drugs rather than to abruptly discontinue use. Salzman concludes that although benzodiazepines are useful and important therapeutic drugs when carefully prescribed and monitored, potential risks must be carefully considered by both physicians and patients.

505   Schneider, Judith Koecheler, Mion, Lorraine C., & Frengley, Dermot J. (January, 1992). Adverse drug reactions in an elderly outpatient population. *American Journal of Hospital Pharmacists, 49*(1), 90-96.

This study investigated the prevalence of adverse drug reactions (ADR) in elderly outpatients, along with factors that might be associated with their occurrence. The medical records of elderly patients attending an interdisciplinary geriatric clinic and a general medical clinic during 1988 were examined for demographic and treatment data and to detect documentation of first-time ADR. The presence of potential drug interactions was also assessed. The sample consisted of 463 patients, of whom 332 attended the medical clinic and 131 attended the geriatric clinic. Potential drug interactions were identified in the records of 143 subjects (31%). There were 107 documented ADR in 97 patients (21%). Of these patients, 86 were noted by the physicians as having had an ADR. Twelve patients were hospitalized as a direct result of an ADR. Significant risk factors for ADR were attendance in the geriatric clinic, the use of potentially harmful drug combinations, and the use of drugs that require therapeutic monitoring. Patient age and the number of drugs had no association with ADR. In the elderly population studied, patients with frailty resulting from multiple pathologies were more likely to have ADR than the healthier elderly, even when physicians simplified their therapeutic regimens.

506   Schroeder, Donna J., & McCart, Gary. (June, 1992). **Exploratory study of medication use in residential-care facilities in San Francisco.** *American Journal of Hospital Pharmacists, 49*(6), 1485-1487.

This study identifies types of medication-related problems present in five residential care facilities in San Francisco that provided living arrangements for the elderly. Medication used by 29 residents in the five residential care facilities was audited. One hundred forty-six medication orders were reviewed (an average of five medications per resident). Each order was screened for accuracy in eight major areas, and a total of 93 medication errors were documented. The observations indicate that medication use in residential care facilities deserves more attention.

507   Semla, Todd P., Cohen, Donna, Paveza, Gregory, Eisdorfer, Carl, Gorelick, Philip, Luchins, Daniel, Hirschman, Robert, Freels, Sally, Levy, Paul, Ashford, J. Wesson, & Shaw, Helen. (1993). **Drug use patterns of persons with Alzheimer's disease and related disorders living in the community.** *Journal of American Geriatrics Society, 41,* 408-413.

This study investigated drug use patterns among persons with Alzheimer's disease, multi-infarct dementia, and mixed Alzheimer's disease and multi-infarct dementia. Subjects were 930 persons in three diagnostic categories, 671 with probable or possible Alzheimer's disease by NINCDS/ADRDA criteria or Alzheimer's disease by DSM-III-R criteria, 162 multi-infarct cases by DSM-III-R criteria, and 97 mixed cases by DSM-III-R criteria. In each diagnostic category, 65% were women, and the majority were ages 70 and over. Data were collected to determine the average number of all prescription and non-prescription drugs and selected therapeutic categories by age, sex, diagnosis, and mini-mental status score at the time of diagnosis or evaluation. Alzheimer patients averaged 2.3 drugs compared with multi-infarct (4.3; p < .0001) and mixed (3.7; p = .0002) patients. The pattern of drug use was different when stratified by therapeutic categories and drug classes. Drug use increased with age, and women used significantly more drugs than men in all three diagnostic categories. Women with Alzheimer's disease used significantly more cardiovascular drugs than men with Alzheimer's disease (p < .05). The lower the Mini-Mental Status score in patients with any dementia, the greater the mean number of central nervous system agents used. The higher the mini-mental status score in a patient with multi-infarct or mixed dementia, the greater the use of cardiovascular drugs. The authors concluded that drug use by Alzheimer patients was lower than in multi-infarct and mixed patients, primarily due to a lower prevalence of cardiovascular drugs.

508   Semla, Todd P., Palla, Kavita, & Poddig, Barbara. (July-August, 1994). Potential impact of OBRA on benzodiazepine and sedative/hypnotic use. *Nursing Home Medicine, 2*(7), 6-18.

The purpose of this retrospective cohort study was to examine to potential impact of the Omnibus Reconciliation Act of 1987 (OBRA) on anxiolytic and sedative/hypnotic prescribing in a 485-bed intermediate care university-affiliated nursing home. The authors reviewed the charts, medication administration records, and computerized pharmacy records of 59 residents who were taking benzodiazepine, other anxiolytic, or sedative/hypnotic in June, 1991. They collected information about diagnoses, indication for use, dose, duration, continuous versus noncontinuous use, and whether the medications had been discontinued or reduced. Of the 59 residents, 98.0% were taking a benzodiazepine and 13.3% were taking a sedative/hypnotic. In 20.0% of cases, the residents were taking more than one of these drugs. Only 12.7% of all residents were taking at least one benzodiazepine or sedative/hypnotic in this study. The authors concluded that the duration and use and continuous dosing seen with these drugs would have often fallen outside of current OBRA guidelines. They believe the major impact of OBRA will be on dosing and duration of use rather than on drug selection.

509   Semla, Todd P., Schwartz, Arthur, Koch, Hugo, & Nelson, Cheryl. (January, 1993). *Patterns of drug prescribing: Vital and health statistics: Health data on older Americans, 1992.* (DHHS Publication No. PHS 93-1411)

The elderly utilize a disproportionate share of health care in general, and drugs in particular. Recent statistics on drug utilization by the elderly indicate that although this group accounts for 12% of the population, they purchase 31% of all prescription drugs sold in the United States each year. The inappropriate prescribing of medications or their misuse can increase the risk of iatrogenic illness and toxicity. These problems are of special concern when dealing with the elderly because of their increased drug use as well as the physiologic consequences of aging and disease on the distribution, metabolism, and elimination of drugs from the body or altered sensitivity to the effects of drugs. A description of drug prescribing patterns in the population ages 55 and over, based on data from the 1985 National Ambulatory Medical Care Survey (NAMCS), is presented. This survey was chosen because of its recent completion and focus on the ambulatory population.

510   Stewart, Ronald B., & Hale, William E. (1992). **Acute confusional states in older adults and the role of polypharmacy.** *Annual Reviews Health, 13,* 412-430.

This review describes problems of acute confusional states resulting from specific drugs, examines the evidence that points to confusional states with polypharmacy, and outlines methods that can be use to prevent the problem. The authors state that cognitive impairment in the elderly represents a major public health problem as the proportion of elderly persons in the population increases. Epidemiologic data show that 1.4% of persons aged 65 to 74 have a dementing illness; this figure rises to 20.8% for persons ages 85 to 89. Acute confusional states (or delirium) differs from Alzheimer's disease by its speed of onset. The patient with acute confusional states may fluctuate between full alertness and coma, and the condition is usually reversible. Acute confusion is a common occurrence among institutionalized elderly persons. In elderly persons, confusional states can be caused by many physical or psychological alterations, including cerebrovascular accidents, seizures, infections, hypoxia, myocardial infarction, depression, and drugs. Polypharmacy, the use of more than one drug to treat symptoms or disease, can be beneficial, but it is often a problem among older persons. The authors offer specific information for preventing problems from occurring.

511   **Suboptimal medication use in the elderly: The tip of the iceberg.
(July 27, 1994).** *Journal of the American Medical Association,*
272(4), 316-317.

The problem of inappropriate prescribing of medications to
older patients is widely acknowledged and has been publicized by
professional societies, governmental organizations, advocacy
groups for the elderly and the media. However, the true
magnitude of the problem remains unclear. In this article the
authors examine the problem by applying explicit criteria defining
inappropriate medication use to data derived from the 1987
National Medical Expenditure Survey. In 1991, two aspects of
medication use were emphasized in designing a criteria:
individual medications or drug categories should be avoided in
nursing home residents except under unusual circumstances and
doses, frequencies, or durations of medication prescriptions
should not be exceeded. A study of 1,106 residents of 12 nursing
homes in the greater Los Angeles, California, area indicated that
40% had at least one inappropriate medication prescription based
on the full list of criteria, which addressed 16 different drug
categories. Findings in this reports confirm the many concerns
about medication use in the elderly.

512   **Thorson, James A., & Thorson, Judy R. J. (1979). Nursing
responsibilities in the administration of drugs to older patients.
In David M. Petersen, Frank J. Whittington, & Barbara P. Payne
(Eds.), *Drugs and the elderly* (pp. 151-161). Springfield, IL:
Charles C. Thomas.**

This chapter discusses the role of the nurse in the
administration of drugs to older patients. The authors point out
that the geriatric patient is often an angry and frustrating person to
deal with and that nurses generally prefer almost any other group
to work with. The authors say that physicians and nurses should
be aware of the social message of medications. While a tranquilizer
is a pill taken by someone who is sick, "A glass of wine, on the
other hand, may have exactly the same effect as the tranquilizer
but conveys the message of wellness and perhaps of sociability or
even celebration." (page 153). They also note that people entering
nursing homes may have developed a dependence on substances
such as alcohol and may suffer withdrawal reactions.

513   *Using your medicines wisely: A guide for the elderly.* **(1980).
Rockville, MD: U. S. Department of Health and Health,
Education and Welfare, Public Health Service, Alcohol, Drug**

Abuse and Mental Health Administration, National Institute on Drug Abuse.

This booklet discusses misuse of prescriptions and over-the-counter drugs and warns that improper use can lead to permanent damage and, in some cases, death.

514 Wade, William E., Cobb, Henry H., III, & Cooper, James W. (Winter, 1986). Drug-related problems in a multiple site ambulatory geriatric population. *Journal of Geriatric Drug Therapy, 1*(2), 67-80.

This study investigated the most prevalent drug-related problems experienced by elderly. Subjects were 52 ambulatory elderly patients in four sites. Data were collected about the patient variables of age, weight, sex, height, number of diagnoses, number of prescriptions, and the number of OTC drugs being taken for possible trends. Data were collected through a series of questions and by examining prescription and OTC medication containers brought by the individual. The most significant drug-related problems found were 1. compliance with directions (19.2%), 2. adverse drug reactions concerning primarily the GI tract (15.4%); and 3. duplication of medication, mainly analgesics (7.7%). Positive correlations were found between the number of diagnoses and age, the number of diagnoses and the numbers of prescription and OTC drugs, and the number of recommendations with the variables of diagnoses, prescription, and OTC drugs.

515 Warner, Joseph J. (November, 1985). Headaches in older patients: Ddx and Tx of common nonvascular causes. *Geriatrics, 40*(11), 69-71, 74-76.

This article discusses headaches in older patients and offers advice in evaluating them for potential causes. Warner states that particular attention should be paid to the possibility of various systemic causes of headache. Therapy for specific headache disorders should be tailored to the individual patient. He recommends considering the patient's overall general, psychological, medical, and neurologic background. The physician must be aware of possible interactions of medications with the therapeutic intervention, as well as possible poor tolerance to specific medications due to preexisting medical or neurologic disorders. A complete history, obtaining information on the temporal pattern of headache, the distribution of pain, and precipitating and alleviating factors, is extremely important in evaluating the elderly patient. A careful physical examination, a neurologic exam, and laboratory investigations may be required prior to making a diagnosis and prescribing treatment.

516 **Weintraub, Michael. (May, 1990). Compliance in the elderly.** *Clinics in Geriatric Medicine, 6*(2), 445–452.

This article discusses issues related to compliance in the elderly with medication regimes. The authors state that compliance in the elderly is approximately equal to that in other patients. However, as a result of sensitivity to medications both in terms of adverse reactions and benefit as well as increased variability and complex medical regimens, a higher level of compliance for elderly people may be necessary. Currently, the data are not adequate to accurately predict either the percentage of medication ingested and the schedule upon which that medication is taken and the reason for those actions. Better data would assist the physician in working with patients and family to increase compliance.

517 **Willcox, Sharon M., Himmelstein, David U., & Woolhandler, Steffie. (July 27, 1994). Inappropriate drug prescribing for the community dwelling elderly.** *Journal of the American Medical Association, 272*(4), 292–296.

This cross-sectional survey investigated the amount of inappropriate drug prescribing for Americans ages 65 and over living in the community. The design was to cross-sectional survey of a national probability sample of older adults. The setting was the 1987 National Medical Expenditure Survey, a national probability sample of United States civilian noninstitutionalized population, with oversampling of some population groups, including the elderly. The subjects were 6,171 people ages 65 and over. The main outcome measure was the incidence of prescribing 20 potentially inappropriate drugs using explicit criteria previously developed by 13 United States and Canadian geriatrics experts. Three cardiovascular drugs identified as potentially inappropriate were analyzed separately since they may be considered appropriate for some noninstitutionalized elderly patients. The results were a total of 23.5% of the subjects received at least one of the 20 contraindicated drugs. While 79.6% of people receiving potentially inappropriate medications received only one such drug, 20.4% received two or more. The most commonly prescribed of these drugs were dipyridamole, propoxyphene, amitriptyline, chlorpropamide, diazepam, indomethacin, and chlordiazepoxide. Including the three controversial cardiovascular agents (propranolol, methyldopa, and reserpine) in the list of contraindicated drugs increased the incidence of probable inappropriate medication use to 32%. The authors concluded was that physicians prescribe potentially inappropriate medications for nearly a quarter of all older people living in the community, placing them at risk of drug adverse effects such as cognitive impairment and sedation. They recommend broader educational and regulatory initiatives to solve the problem.

518 **Williams, Susan G., & DiPalma, Jack A. (January-February, 1992). Medication-induced digestive system injury in the elderly.** *Geriatric Nursing, 13*(1), 39-42.

This review discusses various medications that may cause problems and outlines measures that nurses can use to predict and avoid adverse occurrences. Gastrointestinal injury from medications occurs often in the geriatric population. It has been estimated that 11% of all adverse reactions reported to the Food and Drug Administration involved the digestive system. The gastrointestinal tract generally ages well, but the normal aging process places older patients at risk of medication injury because of polydrug use, changes in distribution and excretion of drugs, metabolism, and sensitivity to certain drugs. Older people tend to have several underlying diseases and take an average of 4.5 drugs daily, increasing the likelihood of adverse drug reactions, because they frequently fail to understand or remember recommended dosage schedules. They may try to save money by sharing medications, and they sometimes lower the dosage to make the drug last longer. Many elderly people discontinue drug usage earlier than advised by their physician such as when symptoms subside or because their medication fails to produce desired results quickly enough. Gastrointestinal reactions and complications associated with medication usage have come to be recognized as frequent health problems for older Americans.

519 **Wolfe, Sondra C., & Schirm, Victoria. (May-June, 1992). Medication counseling for the elderly: Effects on knowledge and compliance after hospital discharge.** *Geriatric Nursing, 13*(3), 134-138.

The purpose of this study was to determine whether hospitalized elderly who receive predischarge medication counseling have more knowledge of and exhibit more compliance with the medication regimen than their uncounseled counterparts. Subjects were 50 people ages 65 and over. The treatment group

(N=25) received counseling and a one-page consumer handout (*The Medication Fact Sheet*) prior to being discharged from the hospital and the control group (N=25) received no counseling. Compliance was defined as the patients' adherence to directions on the prescription container label. Subjects in the treatment group showed significant differences in knowledge of medications as compared to the control group. There was no significant difference between the groups regarding compliance.

520   Yamanaka-Yuen, Nancy A. (1993). Chapter 14: Principles of ethanol drug interactions. In Philip D. Hanston & John R. Horn (Eds.), *Drug interactions and updates* (pp. 89-93). Vancouver, WA: Applied Therapeutics Inc.

This chapter provides a general overview of potential interactions between alcohol and drugs and organizes these interactions into three categories: 1. pharmacodynamic, 2. disulfiram-type, and 3. alteration in drug disposition. Each category is reviewed briefly and is followed by a table which provides specific examples and comments regarding the drugs cited. Some drugs may interact with alcohol through several mechanisms and therefore appear in more than one table. In Category 1 interactions, the effects of alcohol are additive with the effects of the interacting drug. They usually involved the central nervous system but can involve the cardiovascular, gastrointestinal, and endocrine systems. Category 2 interactions can produce an antabuse reaction. Effects include facial flushing, hypotension, nausea, and vomiting. If a large amount of alcohol is ingested with drugs in this group, seizures, arrhythmias, circulatory failure and death may occur. Category 3 interactions changes the way drugs are metabolized. In some cases, the effect could be increased drug toxicity. The chapter includes tables for each interaction category listing drugs, effects and suggested decreases in alcohol intake. For some drugs, the author suggests limiting alcohol intake; for others she recommends abstinence.

521   Walker, Bonnie L. (1984). *Med-ed for seniors* [videotape]. Crofton, MD: Bonnie Walker & Associates, Inc.

This 20-minute video featuring a talk by pharmacist Madeline Feinberg presents information to elderly and their family about talking to doctors, talking to pharmacists, drug side effects, drug interactions, and how to take medications safely.

522 Ziance, Ronald J. (1979). Side effects of drugs in the elderly. In
     David M. Petersen, Frank J. Whittington, & Barbara P. Payne
     (Eds.), *Drugs and the elderly* (pp. 53-79). Springfield, IL: Charles
     C. Thomas.

   The purpose of this article is to alert health care providers
about the serious side effects of prescription and non-prescription
drugs in elderly population. Drugs often involved are
cardiovascular drugs including antihypertensive drugs, diuretics,
and cardiac glycosides. The author also discusses effects of over-
the-counter analgesic drugs such as salicylates. He warns that
"ingestion of ethyl alcohol increases the gastrointestinal bleeding
produced by salicylates; thus this problem is not to be overlooked
in the geriatric population, which consumes a larger volume of
alcoholic beverages than is generally believed." (p. 69)

12

Motor Vehicle Crashes and Pedestrian Accidents

Motor vehicle crashes are the leading cause of accidental death for people between ages 55 and 79. For people between ages 55 and 74, automobile accidents cause more fatalities than all other injuries combined. After age 84, fatalities from motor vehicle crashes drop off sharply and falls become the leading cause of accidental death. Elderly people are also at risk for injury when they are pedestrians. For both crashes and pedestrian accidents, use of alcohol is a major risk factor. Use of medications and declining cognitive and psychomotor abilities are also often involved. Preventing motor vehicle crashes and fatalities is not as easily amenable to interventions as other types of injuries. A great deal of research in this area has been sponsored by the American Automobile Association (AAA) Foundation for Traffic Safety. This chapter includes journal articles and other publications which provide information about the prevalence, risk factors, hazards, and prevention of these injuries.

523   Atkins, R. M., Turner, W. H., Duthie, R. B., & Wilde, B. R. (December 3, 1988). Injuries to pedestrians in road traffic accidents. *British Medical Journal, 297*(6661), 1431-1434.
       This British two-year prospective study examined injuries to pedestrians in road traffic accidents. Subjects were 500 men and women at the accident department of an Oxford, England hospital during 1983 and 1984. Death rates for pedestrians were significantly higher than those inside the cars or riding

motorcycles. The most important factors influencing the seriousness of injuries and deaths were the weight of the vehicle involved in the accident, and the age of the victim. Head injuries were the most common, usually involving a brief concussion. The most common serious injuries were leg injuries. Young children and the elderly made up the majority of accident victims in the study. The authors conclude that pedestrians are at higher risk for admission to the hospital, serious injury, or death than those riding motorcycles or riding in cars, and recommend that further studies investigate ways to reduce this trend.

524   Baker, Susan P., Robertson, Leon S., & O'Neill, Brian. (April, 1974). Fatal pedestrian collisions: Driver negligence. *American Journal of Public Health, 64*(4), 318-325.

The authors studied 180 fatal collisions with Baltimore pedestrians. Referees who reviewed the cases judged 46% of the drivers to be probably negligent, 37% probably not negligent, and 17% negligence unknown. Driver negligence was associated with a history of poor driving. Study drivers also had more points for traffic convictions than the average Maryland driver. The study also found that the pedestrians most likely to be killed are often those whose behavior puts them at risk. It was found that three-fourths of all pedestrians were either under the influence of alcohol, ages 10 and under, or ages 65 and over. The authors suggest that modifying roads, vehicles, and traffic patterns, as well as increasing the legal ramifications of negligent driving may reduce the number of pedestrian deaths and injuries.

525   Ball, Karlene, & Owsley, Cynthia. (October, 1991). Identifying correlates of accident involvement for the older driver. *Human Factors, 33*(5), 583-595.

The authors discuss issues involved with identifying the factors which influence whether older adults drive safely or dangerously. The article explains the conceptual and methodological issues involved, describes why previous research has been unsuccessful, presents a way to approach new research, and recommends new research using large samples. Self-regulation is often flawed because older drivers have little insight into their vision problems. It is also difficult to link age-related deficits and driving accidents. The authors suggest that a prospective study including a training intervention could more accurately examine the difference between the factors that predict accidents and the factors which ultimately cause the accidents.

526   Barr, Robin A. (October, 1991). Recent changes in driving among older adults. *Human Factors, 33*(5), 597-600.
       The author examined driving statistics comparing elderly drivers (ages 65 and over) with all drivers during 1980 and 1989. In that time, despite a drop in the total number of driver deaths (down 8.4%), older driver deaths increased substantially (up 43%). Analyses of population size, numbers of licensed drivers, estimates of miles driven, and crash rates implies that the increase in older driver deaths may be associated with the increasing numbers of licensed elderly drivers and the elderly's increased likelihood of fatality following a motor vehicle crash.

527   Brouwer, Wiebo H., Waterink, Wim, Van Wolffelaar, Peter C., & Rothengatter, Talib. (October, 1991). Divided attention in experienced young and older drivers: Lane tracking and visual analysis in a dynamic driving simulator. *Human Factors, 33*(5), 573-582.
       The authors examined the visual capabilities of older drivers compared to younger drivers. Subjects were 12 healthy young (mean age 26.1 years) and 12 healthy older (mean age 64.4 years) experienced and currently active drivers. The subjects were given a simulated driving task requiring the execution of two continuous visual tasks. The first task was a compensatory land-tracking task, and the second task was a timed, self-paced visual analysis task. The older drivers showed a significantly decreased ability to divide attention, evidenced by their lane tracking and accuracy of visual analysis. The author suggests that this difficulty may be an important factor affecting poor dual-task performance in older drivers.

528   Copeland, Arthur R. (April, 1989). Traffic fatalities among the elderly population: The Metro Dade County experience from 1981-1983. *Medicine, Science and the Law, 29*(2), 159-161.
       The author studied traffic fatalities among elderly victims (ages 65 and older) in Metropolitan Dade County, Florida during 1981 to 1983. The cases were analyzed by age, race, sex, cause of death, and blood alcohol content of the victim. The nature of the accident, the fault, the role of the victim, use of seatbelts, and the reason for the accident were also examined. During this period, 20.6% (251) of the 1,218 traffic-related deaths in Metropolitan Dade County were ages 65 and over. The most common cause of death was multiple injuries. Nearly half of the elderly victims were pedestrians (49.8%), a rate much higher than the national average.

The author estimates that the elderly person is at fault approximately one-third of the time, and suggests that human error is the leading factor in these deaths. Alcohol played a minor role, at best, while crossing the street carelessly and failure to observe right-of-way were major factors.

529   Cushman, Laura A. (August, 1992). *The impact of cognitive decline and dementia on driving in older adults.* Washington, DC: AAA Foundation for Traffic Safety.

This study assessed the ways that visual, cognitive, and driver knowledge measures relate to actual driving performance in a sample of 17 drivers ages 57 to 97. Of the subjects, eight were referred because of suspected early dementia, and nine were self-referred or volunteers. Subjects' driving performance was not associated with reason for referral, age, or sex. The eight drivers who failed to meet the criteria of the assessment were more likely to drive fewer miles, to use compensations while driving (such as avoiding backing up or driving more slowly), to score significantly lower on driver knowledge tests and cognitive measures. After six months, only one of the eight drivers who failed to meet assessment criteria was still driving. Of the nine subjects driving after six months, two had increased their use of driving compensations, and one had decreased his driving to only once a month. The authors suggest that the screening devices used in this study could form the basis for an accurate method of assessing older drivers' ability.

530   DeJoy, David M. (Fall, 1989). An attribution theory perspective on alcohol-impaired driving. *Health Education Quarterly, 16*(3), 359-372.

The author examined previous studies of alcohol-impaired driving to determine whether the attributed responsibility for this behavior varied, and if so, with which variables. Perceptions of the seriousness, responsibility, negligence, and resulting sanctions of alcohol-impaired driving were associated with the consequences produced, rather than from the behavior itself. In other words, alcohol-impaired driving was not perceived as serious or negligent unless the results caused harm to others. Impaired driving situations were also not seen as personally relevant. Consumption of alcohol before driving was not seen as a problem if consumption did not exceed legal limits. Those with a history of alcohol-impaired driving had a less serious perception of impaired driving than others. The author suggests that these studies may have practical applications in already-existing efforts to curb alcohol-impaired driving, and may perhaps give some insight as to the reasons for and reactions to this behavior.

531   *Drivers 55 plus: Check your own performance.* (1994). Washington, DC: AAA Foundation for Traffic Safety.

This book contains a self-rating test and feedback for older drivers to create awareness of their own driving ability. The test includes a rating guide to compute the score, and rate the person's level of safe or unsafe driving. The rest of the book contains discussion of the safe and unsafe driving practices on the test, and gives safety tips to help the older driver drive safely.

532   Eisenhandler, Susan A. (1990). The asphalt identikit: Old age and the driver's license. *International Journal of Aging and Human Development, 30*(1), 1-14.

The author discusses the "asphalt identikit," a valid driver's license and the ability to drive, which can be vital to an elderly person. The author interviewed a sample of 50 elderly men and women (ages 62 and over). The subjects were resistant and defiant about the prospect of losing their licenses, while freely admitting that vision and health problems made them restrict their driving. Because having a driver's license and driving are symbols of identity, independence, and connection to the mainstream, the older driver may resist giving up driving, even when he or she is no longer able to drive safely.

533   Fell, James C., & Nash, Carl E. (Fall, 1989). The nature of the alcohol problem in U. S. fatal crashes. *Health Education Quarterly, 16*(3), 335-344.

The authors discuss alcohol-related traffic fatalities between 1982 and 1987. Alcohol-related fatalities during these years declined, mostly due to increased public awareness, tougher laws, better enforcement of laws, an increase in the legal drinking age, public and private prevention programs, socioeconomic factors, and demographic factors. The reduction in fatalities was significant among teenagers, females, drivers surviving an accident, teenage pedestrians, older drivers, and drivers in daytime crashes. Despite this drop in fatalities, an estimated 23,630 people were killed in alcohol-related crashes during 1987. The authors recommend that further efforts like those influencing the 1982 to 1987 drop in fatalities will determine the degree to which these deaths will decrease in the future.

534   Gresset, Jacques, & Meyer, François. (July-August, 1994). Risk of automobile accidents among elderly drivers with impairments or chronic diseases. *Canadian Journal of Public Health, 85*(4), 282-285.

The authors conducted a case-control study in Quebec to document the risk of road accidents associated with impairments or chronic medical conditions. Case subjects were 1,400 drivers who reported having an accident with either mild bodily injury or only property damage during their 70th year in 1988 and 1989. Control subjects were 2,636 drivers of the same age. The study included any medical conditions, as well as driving habits and mileage. The results suggested that elderly drivers with impairments or chronic medical conditions were not at increased risk of road accidents. Only those with arrhythmia had a significant increase in risk. The authors suggest that these results indicate a need to reevaluate the norms currently in place for elderly drivers.

535   Hart, Robert P., Colenda, Christopher C., & Hamer, Robert M. (January, 1991). Effects of buspirone and alprazolam on the cognitive performance of normal elderly subjects. *American Journal of Psychiatry, 148*(1), 73-78.

The authors studied cognitive disability related to the behavioral side effects of medications given for anxiety (such as benzodiazepines) by evaluating the memory/learning and speed effects of doses of buspirone, a non-benzodiazepine, and alprazolam, a benzodiazepine. Subjects were 60 healthy elderly (ages 62 and over) who were assigned to one of three groups. After two days, subjects were given one of the drugs or a placebo (sugar pill) for 14 days. Behavioral assessment included recall memory for word lists, retention of pictures over one hour, and a questionnaire asking subjects about their mood. The results showed that buspirone did not affect reaction time, speed, or memory function, and that alprazolam had minimal effects; however, the effects of either drug on less healthy elderly are unknown.

536   Jette, Alan M., & Branch, Laurence G. (February, 1992). A ten year follow-up of driving patterns among the community-dwelling elderly. *Human Factors, 34*(1), 25-31.

This study used Massachusetts Health Care Panel Study data to examine age-related changes in driving patterns over a 10-year period. Subjects were a group of 1,625 community-dwelling elderly (ages 65 and over). In 1974, 86% of men and 76% of women used a car as their main transportation. At each follow-up, 87% of those who had relied on a car at the start of the study continued to rely on the car. Approximately 75% or more of those who were self-reliant in driving a car at each assessment were still self-reliant at the subsequent follow-up. The authors suggest that these prospective data indicate that a large proportion of American elderly continue to rely on the car and to drive into their eighties and nineties. This further suggests that, as the elderly population increases, there will be more elderly drivers. Those who stopped driving tended to do so for reasons of declining health or increasing disability, which suggests that self-regulation of driving may effectively decrease the number of at-risk elderly drivers on the road.

537 Kaszniak, Alfred W., Keyl, Penelope M., & Albert, Marilyn S. (October, 1991). Dementia and the older driver. *Human Factors*, *33*(5), 527-537.

The authors reviewed the available research on dementia and driving and discussed issues that must be considered in attempting to apply this developing body of research to practical problems, such as the relicensing process for selected drivers. The research, though sparse and problematic, indicates that Alzheimer's disease and other dementia patients are at increased risk for motor vehicle crashes and getting lost while driving than others the same age. The author suggests that four areas for future research may help improve dementia patients' road safety: defining the relationship of neurophysical characteristics to driving history and performance, developing standards for assessing driving ability, determining the subjects' awareness of their driving limitations, and, for those getting lost or confused, investigating more advanced electronics that could provide vehicle guidance.

538 Klein, Ronald. (October, 1991). Age-related eye disease, visual impairment, and driving in the elderly. *Human Factors*, *33*(5), 521-525.

The author reviewed the relationship of age-related eye diseases and visual problems and driving. Decline in vision can be partially connected to an increase in vehicular accidents for every mile driven by elderly people. Four age-related eye diseases — cataract, macular degeneration, open-angle glaucoma, and diabetic retinopathy — are primarily responsible for the decline in visual acuity and visual field in the elderly. Few epidemiological data are available about these diseases, and at present they are not preventable. The author recommended further study on visual decline and how it affects driving performance, and on practical ways to identify and assess the visually at-risk elderly driver.

539   Kline, Donald. (March, 1991). *Aging and the visibility of highway signs: A new look through old eyes.* Washington, DC: AAA Foundation for Traffic Safety.

This report describes a research program to understand and improve the effects of visual aging on the visibility of highway signs. The studies compared age-related differences on visibility, evaluated the degree to which the visibility of highway signs could be improved for all age groups, and determined whether the visibility differences between all age groups could be duplicated through image-processing techniques. Symbolic signs were visible at much greater distances than text signs for all three age groups, especially in darker conditions. There was significant variation between the comprehension of different signs. Standard symbolic highway signs offer drivers about twice as much time to respond to them as text signs. According to the study, a "low pass" design approach, one that uses fewer high-contrast details, can produce marked improvements in the visibility of standard symbolic highway signs for drivers of any age. The findings also demonstrate that contrast sensitivity testing used with image-processing techniques (such as filters and lighting) can be used to assess the impact of visual aging on highway signs.

540   Malfetti, James L., & Winter, Darlene J. (1990). *A graded license for special older drivers: Premise and guidelines.* Washington, DC: AAA Foundation for Traffic Safety.

The authors describe their study about and final guidelines for a program of graded licenses for older drivers. Their premise is that a total revocation of driving privileges is often unnecessary, and that a system of grading licenses according to the older drivers' individual limitations would allow those who are able to drive safely under certain conditions to continue driving. The study consisted of several focus groups, discussion groups, and a Delphi method opinion poll of experts. The guidelines were developed from the study and from relevant literature on the subject, and range from improving older drivers' perception of the licensing department, identifying the candidates for graded licenses, developing a standard set of conditions, implementing the program, and evaluating the effectiveness of the program. The authors suggest that a graded license system could help improve quality of life for those who would otherwise have their licenses revoked.

541   Malfetti, James L., & Winter, Darlene J. (1991). *Concerned about an older driver?* Washington, DC: AAA Foundation for Traffic Safety.

This book is a guide for the friends and families of older drivers. The authors describe ways to assess an older driver, including self-assessment, vision and medical examinations, checking medications taken, and observing road performance. If the assessment reveals driving problems, there are several ways to help: older driver improvement courses, programs from licensing agencies, graded licenses, and alternative transportation. The authors also review age-related changes that affect driving, such as vision, hearing, and decision-making.

542   Marottoli, Richard A., Ostfeld, Adrian M., Merrill, Susan S., Perlman, Gary D., Foley, Daniel J., & Cooney, Leo M., Jr. (1993). Driving cessation and changes in mileage driven among elderly individuals. *Journals of Gerontology, 48*(5), S255-S261.

This study examined the factors which influenced community-dwelling elderly to stop driving or to decrease the number of miles they drove. Of 1,331 elderly subjects (ages 65 and older) who completed the driving survey, 456 were still driving, 309 had stopped driving, and 566 had never driven during 1983 to 1989. The individual factors influencing those who had stopped driving included higher age, lower income, not working, neurologic disease, cataracts, lower level of physical activity, and functional disability. If none of these factors were present, none of the subjects stopped driving. If one or two factors were present, 17% stopped, and if three or more factors were present, 49% stopped. High mileage drivers (5,000 or more miles per year) were more likely young, male, and still working. Among those subjects still driving in 1989, 42% reported driving fewer miles. Reducing mileage was associated with increasing age and disability. An understanding of the factors which influence the elderly to stop or limit their driving will help identify high-risk drivers in this population.

543   Mayer, David L., & Laux, Lila F. (September, 1992). *Evaluating vehicle displays for older drivers.* Washington, DC: AAA Foundation for Traffic Safety.

The authors studied the instrument panels of 1990 model cars. There were three major types of displays: traditional analog, bar graph, and readout. There has been little systematic examination of the differences in speed, ease and accuracy of use of these various types of displays. The study used 12 computer displays designed to simulate current instrument panels. Subjects were 60 active drivers ranging in age from 20 to 80, who had to maintain performance on a demanding tracking task that simulated driving while also watching a cluster of four displays. On the no-color displays, the older subjects made more tracking errors, and were slower to respond to the displays than younger subjects. All subjects responded faster when color was added to the displays. Adding dynamic color to the displayed eliminated the age-related decrease in reaction time. The authors suggest that future design of instrument panels include research on what features can minimize or eliminate the age-related changes in sensory perception and reaction time.

544   McPherson, Kenard, Ostrow, Andrew, & Shaffron, Peter. (June, 1989). *Physical fitness and the aging driver.* Washington, DC: AAA Foundation for Traffic Safety.

This case-control study examines the relationship between physical fitness and the performance of older drivers. Subjects were 36 elderly men and women (ages 60 and over). Case subjects took a range-of-motion exercise program at home before driving. They were also taught to use breathing and relaxation techniques to lower their perceived stress while driving. All subjects received range-of-motion assessments, an anxiety assessment, reaction time tests, and field-assessment of driving skills. Findings include the following: that range-of-motion training improved the subjects' trunk rotation and shoulder flexibility, that stress management training lowered driver anxiety in stressful driving situations, and that stress management training did not improve reaction time, movement, or handling skills, but did improve observation skills. The authors recommend further study on the effects of exercise and stress management on driving skills in this population.

545   Miller, Denver J., & Morley, John E. (July, 1993). Attitudes of physicians toward elderly drivers and driving policy. *Journal of the American Geriatrics Society, 41*(7), 722-724.

The authors examined physicians' attitudes toward and knowledge about older drivers. Physician members of the American Geriatrics Society (n=5,009) were asked to complete a questionnaire exploring their practice, record keeping, how often they educated, counseled, and reported patients to authorities when appropriate, and their own understanding of driving issues and physician responsibilities in their state. The survey produced a 48% response rate. There was no consensus among physicians, who showed a broad range of attitudes and practices. The respondents generally believed that they had a legal responsibility, but were uncertain about how to assess driving ability and their responsibility toward older drivers. The authors suggest that physicians should be aware there are resources available to aid in the assessment and evaluation of older drivers. Physicians should also consider giving their patients referrals to driver refresher courses.

546   *Older driver skill assessment and resource guide.* (1992). **Washington, DC: American Association of Retired Persons.**
      This handbook on driving for older people contains a series of exercises and questions to help assess driving skills. Some of the subjects discussed are reaction time, distractions, what safety features to look for on an automobile, vision, and accidents. After the assessment, the reader should be able to evaluate his or her driving skills, and decide what (if any) action is necessary. The book also gives safety tips and telephone numbers for state agencies where older drivers may get resource materials for this subject.

547   **Panek, Paul E., & Rearden, John J. (September, 1987). Age and gender effects on accident types for rural drivers.** *Journal of Applied Gerontology, 6*(3), 332-346.
      This study classified different types of accidents among rural drivers, and examined whether these accidents differed by age and gender. Data were taken from 12 months of police reports in a daily newspaper serving a rural midwestern area. Accidents were categorized as laterally moving vehicle, following, gap acceptance, laterally moving object, intruding approach, passing, tracking, skidding, or attention deficit. These types are described in the article, along with examples of each. Those determined to be at fault were grouped by age. The results indicated that men had significantly more following and skidding accidents, and that women had significantly more intruding–approach accidents. The

authors also found that age was associated with laterally moving vehicle and attention-deficit accidents, that all age groups were likely to have intruding-approach accidents, and that following and skidding accidents generally decreased with age.

548   Parasuraman, Raja, & Nestor, Paul. (May, 1993). Attention and driving: Assessment in elderly individuals with dementia. *Clinics in Geriatric Medicine, 9*(2), 377-387.

The authors discuss various assessments to determine driving ability in older drivers with dementia. The crash risk for these drivers is currently not assessed, except for vision tests and other measures aimed at drivers without dementia. Assessment of attention is important in the elderly population, and especially in the elderly with dementia. Because attention, especially when divided or distracted, is important to driving skills, dementia-related compromises in attention should be included in any assessment of older drivers. The authors recommend that attention tests should be added to already existing measures of driving skill for this population.

549   Parasuraman, Raja & Nestor, Paul G. (October, 1991). Attention and driving skills in aging and Alzheimer's disease. *Human Factors, 33*(5), 539-557.

The author reviewed current literature on the relationship of dementia to driving skills, and recommends that license renewal be based on driving competence, not on chronological age or medical diagnosis. Current licensing procedures, even with a road test, do not adequately evaluate the attention factors impaired by dementia that are important to safe driving. The author suggests that driver training programs which help improve attention and other cognitive skills should be developed and made available for all older drivers, especially those with dementia.

550   Pedestrian fatalities — New Mexico, 1958-1987. (May 17, 1991). *Morbidity and Mortality Weekly Report, 40*(19), 312-314.

A study of New Mexico pedestrian fatalities during a 30-year period showed that rates of fatalities were significantly different between genders and ethnic groups. Rates of pedestrian fatalities were higher for males than for females, and higher for American Indians (in all age groups) than for other groups. Because minorities, especially those in lower socioeconomic groups, are disproportionately represented in injuries, the article suggests that systems used to track the prevalence and causes of injury include ethnic data.

551   Persson, Diane. (1993). The elderly driver: Deciding when to stop. *The Gerontologist, 33*(1), 88-91.

The author describes a study examining an elderly person's decision to stop driving, and the role that physicians and family play in this decision. Subjects were 56 elderly recruited from retirement communities (ages 66 and over) who had stopped driving. Most of the subjects (84%) felt that they stopped driving at an appropriate time. Reasons given for the decision to stop driving included the advice of a doctor, feeling nervous while driving, having trouble seeing, medical conditions, advice from family or friends, impaired coordination, finances, minor accidents, and a revoked license. Physicians, family, and friends had a limited influence on the subjects' decision to stop driving. The results suggest that older drivers believe that the decision to stop is a personal decision, and that physician or family intervention should be used as a last resort. The author recommends that older drivers be educated about the factors that may affect their driving as they age.

552   Ray, Wayne A., Fought, Randy L., & Decker, Michael D. (October 1, 1992). Psychoactive drugs and the risk of injurious motor vehicle crashes in elderly drivers. *American Journal of Epidemiology, 136*(7), 873-883.

This retrospective cohort study examined motor vehicle crashes to determine whether commonly-prescribed psychoactive drugs increased the risk of these crashes. Data were obtained from the Tennessee Medicaid program, driver's license files, and police reports of injurious crashes. Subjects were 16,262 Medicaid enrollees ages 65 to 84 who had a valid driver's license during the study period (1984 to 1988). The four groups of psychoactive drugs studied were benzodiazepines, cyclic antidepressants, oral opioid analgesics, and antihistamines. For those currently using psychoactive drugs, the risk of being involved in an injury-causing crash was significantly increased. Those using one or more benzodiazepines, one or more cyclic antidepressants, or, in some cases, a combination of the two were at higher risk for crashes, a risk that grew in relation to the dosage. The authors suggest that the disorders treated by these medications may also be a factor in these crashes, and that future research should be done in this area.

553   Ray, Wayne A., Gurwitz, Jerry, Decker, Michael D., & Kennedy,
       Dianne L. (February, 1992). Medications and the safety of the
       older driver: Is there a basis for concern? *Human Factors, 34*(1),
       33-47.
           The authors reviewed the effects of certain medications on
       driving ability in the elderly. Medications that affect the central
       nervous system, including benzodiazepines, antihistamines, cyclic
       antidepressants, narcotic analgesics, and hypoglycemics, may
       impair driving. Research on these medications in younger drivers
       have shown impaired performance and an increased risk of motor
       vehicle crashes. Even though the elderly frequently take these
       drugs and are more susceptible to their effects on the central
       nervous system, there are no direct data indicating whether or not
       medications adversely affect driving safety in this population,
       research which is greatly needed.

554   Reduction in alcohol-related traffic fatalities—United States,
       1990-1992. (December 3, 1993). *Morbidity and Mortality Weekly
       Report, 42*(47), 905-909.
           Alcohol-related motor vehicle crashes are a leading cause of
       unintentional injury deaths and a substantial contributor to health-
       care costs in the United States. This report summarizes data
       regarding alcohol-related traffic fatalities from the National
       Highway Traffic Safety Administration's (NHTSA) Fatal Accident
       Reporting System during 1982 to 1992. The findings suggest that
       current programs to reduce the rate of alcohol-related driving are
       successful. Future campaigns from the NHTSA will combine
       issues related to impaired driving and failure to use seatbelts.

555   Retchin, Sheldon M., & Anapolle, Jackie. (May, 1993). An
       overview of the older driver. *Clinics in Geriatric Medicine, 9*(2),
       279-296.
           This article describes the older driver, including data on
       traffic violations, crash rates, and fatalities. Because of the
       increasing dependence on the car for principal transportation and
       the increasing the number of elderly in America, there are now
       more drivers ages 65 and over than ever. Research suggests that
       skills needed to drive safely are compromised in later years.
       Cognitive impairment, psychomotor slowing, reduced strength,
       vision problems, and life changes can all impair the older driver.
       Most states have policies to evaluate and identify older drivers at
       risk for crashes. These policies have legal and ethical

complications, because they involve issues of public safety, independence, and liability, especially for physicians.

556   Roberts, W. Neal, & Roberts, Pamela C. (May, 1993). Evaluation of the elderly driver with arthritis. *Clinics in Geriatric Medicine,* *9*(2), 311-322.

The authors discuss the motor vehicle crash risks associated with osteoarthritis. Because the decreased level of flexibility and increased joint pain affect the driver's ability to grip the steering wheel, brake, and perform other driving maneuvers, the authors suggest a five-minute, eight point screening examination to determine the level of the arthritis patient's driving impairment. Patients with arthritis can also have perceptual defects, cognitive changes, and psychosocial problems in conjunction with the arthritis. These factors, along with the effects of arthritis medication, should also be evaluated in the older driver. Many arthritis sufferers can continue to drive safely with proper treatment and the aid of modified controls in the car, many of which are widely available and inexpensive. Power steering and automatic transmission are the most helpful of these devices.

557   Rosenbloom, Sandra. (May, 1993). Transportation needs of the elderly population. *Clinics in Geriatric Medicine, 9*(2), 297-310.

The author reviews the transportation needs and problems of the elderly. Because a majority of elderly people are dependent on cars for transportation because of their proximity to health care and other needed services, the older person's ability to drive can be a crucial factor in their quality of life and continued health. Because public and specialized transportation programs are still too limited to compensate for the mobility lost as a result of not driving, many elderly have limited access to medical care and social programs. The author recommends that transportation planners reevaluate their programs to include more flexibility and access for the elderly.

558   Safety restraint assessment—Iowa, 1987-1988. (November 3, 1989). *Morbidity and Mortality Weekly Report, 38*(43), 735-743.

The 1,454 non-fatally injured car accident victims in the state of Iowa who were brought to 16 hospitals for emergency medical assistance during a five-month period were included in a study of safety-restraint devices. This population was approximately 20% of all individuals injured in similar crashes during this period. Of this group, 697 (48%) were determined to have been wearing seatbelts at the time of the accident. Those who were not using seatbelts were most likely to be male, younger, having used alcohol and driving at speeds in excess of 55 miles per hour. These individuals were hospitalized three times as often as individuals who wore seatbelts. They were also 8.4 times more vulnerable to head injuries with loss of consciousness. Unbelted victims of car accidents sustained 2.7 times more fractures and were 2.8 times more likely to have a cut or laceration. The average hospital cost of caring for an unbelted person was $2,462, compared with the statistically lower bill of $753 for those wearing seatbelt restraints. Instruction on the importance of wearing a seatbelt for children and education of the older more risk prone 16- to 25-year-old population concerning alcohol, excessive speed and the use of restraints will be required to reduce the rate of accidents and injury.

559   Schiff, William, & Oldak, Rivka. (February, 1993). *Functional screening of older drivers using interactive computer-video scenarios*. Washington, DC: AAA Foundation for Traffic Safety.

The authors examined the effectiveness of using computer simulations to assess driving ability, especially in older drivers. Subjects were 170 drivers between ages 17 and 91 from various sites in the United States. Computer-video driving tasks and questionnaires recorded their functional driving ability, medical status, driving habits, and accident records. The results indicate that this 15-minute assessment had a high degree of success and user satisfaction. The authors suggest that this kind of brief assessment should be further refined, and eventually used in many different settings such as auto clubs, hospitals, or driving schools.

560   *Safety belt sense*. (November, 1983). Gaithersburg, MD: National Institute on Aging.

This pamphlet explains the advantages of wearing seatbelts with a specific focus on older adults. The author describes the safety benefits of seatbelts, and disputes some of the reasons often given for not wearing a seatbelt.

561   Shinar, David, & Schieber, Frank. (October, 1991). Visual requirements for safety and mobility of older drivers. *Human Factors, 33*(5), 507-519.

The authors describe the issues associated with the vision problems of older drivers. Because vision is important to safe driving, and because vision deteriorates with age, adequate and accurate assessment and treatment of vision problems affecting driving is essential. The authors suggest that visual training, along with environmental and vehicle modifications can help the older driver compensate for any vision problems that could impair their ability to drive. The authors recommend further research in this area.

562 Sleet, David A., Sheard, Judith, Lavelle, Judith, Hartigan, Phyllis & Yee, Stefanie. (Fall, 1989). Resource guide to alcohol-impaired driving programs and materials. *Health Education Quarterly, 16*(3), 439-447.

This article describes the various alcohol-impaired driving prevention programs and resources available through government agencies, computer on-line services, and private foundations. The article includes a list of these organizations, with addresses, phone numbers, and information about each organization.

563 Smith, Perry F., Remington, Patrick L., & the Behavioral Risk Factor Surveillance Group. (Fall, 1989). The epidemiology of drinking and driving: Results from the behavioral risk factor surveillance system, 1986. *Health Education Quarterly, 16*(1), 345-358.

The authors studied drinking and driving among 34,395 randomly selected subjects from 28 states. The subjects were asked questions about their drinking habits, drinking and driving, smoking habits, use of smokeless tobacco, use of seatbelts, and demographic information. In this sample, 4.1% reported drinking and driving at least once in the month before the interview. Among those who reported having at least one drink in the previous month, 7.2% reported drinking and driving during that month. Men reported more drinking and driving than women. Those aged 18 to 24 and 25 to 34 reported the highest level of drinking and driving. Whites had a higher prevalence of drinking and driving than other ethnic groups. Other demographics, such as marital status and income, also influenced prevalence of drinking and driving. The results also showed that other risk behaviors, such as smoking and failure to wear seatbelts, were also associated with drinking and driving. The authors caution that these data, because they were based on self-report interviews, may underestimate the actual level of drinking and driving.

564   Staplin, Loren, & Fisk, Arthur D. (October, 1991). A cognitive engineering approach to improving signalized left–turn intersections. *Human Factors, 33*(5), 559-571.

This study evaluated age-related differences in drivers' deciding whether or not it is safe to turn at a signalized intersection. Younger (mean age 37 years) and older (mean age 71 years) drivers were tested at simulating intersections. Subjects were asked to decide as quickly as possible whether they had the right-of-way to make a left turn. The first study used signals only, and the second study combined signals with other variables found in real-life situations. Advance notice of the rules for right-of-way decisions improved the accuracy of decisions for all groups. To accommodate older drivers, the authors cautioned against the use of signals that must be interpreted differently than previous experience has dictated.

565   Stelmach, George, & Nahom, Ariella. (February, 1992). Cognitive-motor abilities of the elderly driver. *Human Factors, 34*(1), 53-65.

The authors reviewed the literature on age-related problems that affect older drivers. Deficits in reaction and movement time are explained in detail, with discussions of possible effects on driving. Research indicates that these deficits may be reversible by retraining, practice, or other type of intervention. Because the research is sparse, the authors recommend that future studies isolate these reaction and movement variables, and evaluate their effects on driving.

566   Stewart, Ronald B., Moore, Mary T., Marks, Ronald G., May, Franklin E., & Hale, William E. (January, 1993). *Driving cessation and accidents in the elderly: An analysis of symptoms, diseases, cognitive dysfunction and medications*. Washington, DC: AAA Foundation for Traffic Safety.

This study comes from the Florida Geriatric Research Program in Dunedin, Florida. The authors used longitudinal health information on 1,470 elderly subjects (ages 55 and over) gathered since 1975 to determine whether the decision to stop driving was associated with specific symptoms, diseases or medications, and to find out whether specific symptoms, diseases or medications were associated with an increase in reported traffic accidents. In this investigation, 20.9% of women and 9.8% of men had stopped driving. Six factors influencing this decision were age, female gender, macular degeneration, stroke, hospitalization in the past year, eye problems, and Parkinsonism. Also, 9.1% of women and 11.2% of men reported a traffic accident in the past five years. Four factors predicted traffic accidents: bursitis, feet or legs cold on exposure to cold, protein in the urine, and irregular heartbeat. Age and gender were not significant factors in predicting traffic accidents in this study, and no specific drug ingredients or therapeutic categories of drugs were associated with traffic accidents.

567 Umansky, Diane. (Winter 1994-1995). **When is it time to give up the car keys?** *Family Safety and Health, 53*(4), 21.

This article presents issues related to elderly drivers. In Illinois, drivers ages 75 to 80 must take a written, visual and road test every four years; those ages 81 to 86 must take these tests every two years; those ages 87 and over must be tested every year. The author lists questions that older drivers could ask themselves which will help them evaluate their driving ability. Among the recommended activities are taking vision tests, wearing a safety belt, and finding out about the effects of medications. The author also offers advice for children with older parents to help them prepare for the time when they may need to give up driving such as choosing a home near family and friends, public transportation, stores, and doctors' offices; near train or bus stations; and in an area where there is free transportation through community centers and churches.

568 Use of seat belts—DeKalb County, Georgia, 1986. (1987). *Morbidity and Mortality Weekly Report, 36*(27), 433-437.

This study examined the use of seatbelts by Georgia residents. Interviews with 337 subjects showed that 38% did not use seatbelts. Prevalence was higher among males, nonwhites, and those with 12 or fewer years of education. Failure to use seatbelts was reported by 44% of those ages 16 to 29, 34% of those ages 30 to 59, and 40% of those ages 60 and over. Compared to non-users, those who used seatbelts were more likely in favor of a mandatory use law, and more likely to recognize the safety value of wearing a seatbelt. The major reasons given for not wearing the seatbelt were traveling a short distance (28%), discomfort (23%), fear of entrapment (13%), unnecessary (9%), and difficult to wear (6%).

569 von Mering, Otto, Donnelly, Michelle, & Kaplan, Holly S. (September-October, 1994). **Driving smart: A quality-of-life issue for elders.** *Aging Today, 15*(5), 12.

The authors describe a University of Florida Center for Gerontological Studies survey on elderly drivers. Of the 1,113 elderly subjects (ages 55 and over) from a local health maintenance organization, 89% reported that they were not ready to stop driving. More than half of the subjects had changed their driving habits recently, avoiding driving at night, or in other risky situations. Walking was not an option for 45% of subjects, who reported living beyond walking distance of necessary services. Improvements in cars and roads, special equipment, and refresher driving classes have helped the elderly drive safely. The authors recommend that improved public transportation may help older people stay independent, even beyond the time when they can no longer drive.

570   **Wallace, Robert B., & Retchin, Sheldon M. (February, 1992). A geriatric and gerontologic perspective on the effects of medical conditions on older drivers: Discussion of Waller.** *Human Factors, 34*(1), 17-24.

This article discusses the article by Julian Waller on the effects of medical conditions on the older driver from a gerontologic and geriatric perspective. The authors caution against assigning any specific age threshold for an enhanced driver testing and certification program. Because the risks for older drivers are not necessarily determined by chronological age, a system of age classification would leave out those at risk for health or other reasons, especially those in younger populations. The authors suggest three approaches for assessment and classification of at-risk drivers: the medical model, where diseases are used as risk factors, the functional status model, where the driver's ability to function as a driver is assessed; and the behavioral model, where emotional illnesses and social vitality are used as risk factors for motor vehicle crashes.

571   **Waller, Julian A. (February, 1992). Research and other issues concerning effects of medical conditions on elderly drivers.** *Human Factors, 34*(1), 3-15.

The author reviewed the available research on the medical problems of older drivers. This research is limited by the omission of seven issues relevant to impaired older drivers: difficulties in diagnostic accuracy, sample size, and sample selection; vague criteria for excessive risk of motor vehicle crashes; the influence of multiple medical conditions; the interaction between the driver and the environment; inadequate screening measures; the influence of age and aging; and the impact of commercial driving. The author discusses medication conditions affecting driving, including, cardiovascular disease, diabetes mellitus, alcoholism, seizures, syncope, and physical frailty, and gives several recommendations for future research on older drivers.

572   Waller, Patricia F. (October, 1991). The older driver. *Human Factors, 33*(5), 499-505.

        The author profiles older drivers, a group that is growing rapidly in a system that is not designed for them. Because older drivers have different needs than younger drivers, and because they are at higher risk for injury and death in motor vehicle crashes, the author recommends that the specific needs and abilities of this age group be studied. The older driver will, at some point, probably need to restrict his or her driving, and perhaps even stop driving, but this does not indicate that highway design should not be improved to accommodate this age group. The author suggests modifying the driving environment where necessary to ensure that older drivers may drive with a reasonable level of safety.

573   Zegeer, Charles, V., Stutts, Jane C., Huang, Herman, Zhou, Mei, & Rodgman, Eric. (January, 1993). Prevention of motor vehicle injuries to elderly pedestrians. *Family and Community Health, 15*(4), 38-56.

        This study analyzed over 26,000 pedestrian-motor vehicle crashes in North Carolina during an 11-year period (1980 to 1990). Pedestrian victims included 1,758 victims ages 65 and over. Similar findings were reported from an analysis of 70,825 fatal pedestrian-motor vehicle crashes occurring nationwide from 1980 to 1989 and identified from the Fatal Accident Reporting System (FARS) database. About 15,000 pedestrians ages 65 and over were killed during 1980 to 1989. Based on these results, the authors give a series of recommendations for intervention programs. Education interventions cautioning the elderly about risks have already been developed by organizations like the American Association of Retired Persons (AARP). Laws concerning jaywalking should be enforced, as well as laws for motorists concerning yielding to pedestrians, running red lights, speeding, and driving drunk. Other ordinances related to parking and bus routes could also help prevent injuries to elderly pedestrians. Road signs for pedestrians, improving sidewalks, careful placement of street furniture (such as poles, benches, or newspaper racks), handrails, adequate signals, pedestrian islands, roadway lighting, over- and under-passes, pedestrian malls, and barriers can all help the elderly pedestrian avoid traffic and walk safely, even in heavy traffic areas.

13

Suicide

The elderly population is disproportionately represented in the number of completed suicides each year. This chapter includes articles and books dealing with suicide prevalence, risk factors, and prevention interventions. Another issue related to the topic which has provoked numerous articles in the literature is the appropriateness of suicide for elderly people who are terminally ill or in pain. This chapter also includes articles which discuss methods of identifying or screening for people with suicide ideation. Because depression is often related to suicide, this section also includes articles on that topic.

574 Beck, Aaron T., Steer, Robert A., Beck, Judith S., & Newman, Cory F. (Summer, 1993). Hopelessness, depression, suicidal ideation, and clinical diagnosis of depression. *Suicide and Life-Threatening Behavior, 23*(2), 139-145.

This study investigated the relevance of a clinical diagnosis of depression for explaining the discrepant relationships of hopelessness and depression with suicidal ideation. The Beck Depression Inventory (BDI) Hopelessness Scale (BHS), and the Scale for Suicide Ideation (SSI) were administered to 1,306 (72%) patients with at least one DSM-III-R mood disorder and 488 (27.3%) patients without any mood disorders. Analysis of the data showed that hopelessness was 1.3 times more important than depression for explaining suicidal ideation. The interactions of the BDI and BHS with diagnostic group were not significant.

575   Beck, Aaron T., Steer, Robert A., & Brown, Gary. (Spring, 1993).
       Dysfunctional attitudes and suicidal ideation in psychiatric
       outpatients. *Suicide and Life-Threatening Behavior*, 23(1), 11-20.
          This study investigated the relationship between specific sets
       of dysfunctional attitudes and suicidal ideation. Beck and his
       colleagues administered the 100-item Dysfunctional Attitude Scale
       (DAS) to 908 psychiatric outpatients along with the Beck
       Depression Inventory (BDI), Hopelessness Scale (BHS), Self-
       Concept Test (BST), and Scale for Suicide Ideation (SSI). They used
       the SSI to classify the outpatients into 97 (10.7%) suicide ideators
       and 811 (89.3%) nonideators. They scored the DAS for nine
       subscales. Data analysis suggested that none of the DAS subscales
       discriminated the ideators after controlling for sex, age, diagnosis
       of a mood or panic disorder, comorbidity, presence of a
       personality disorder, a history of past suicide attempt, the BHI, the
       BHS, and the BST. History of past suicide attempt and
       hopelessness overshadowed the contributions of sets of
       dysfunctional attitudes for identifying and explaining suicidal
       ideation.

576   Blazer, Dan. (1991). Suicide risk factors in the elderly: An
       epidemiological study. *Journal of Geriatric Psychiatry*, 24(2), 175-
       190.
          This article is a review of epidemiological data relevant to
       the association of age and death by suicide including a review of
       the interaction of age and other known risk factors for suicide.
       Blazer examined period effects and cohort effects and found that
       both had an impact on suicide rates. Other risk factors include sex,
       race, marital status, and biochemical factors. The author concludes
       that age alone cannot be eliminated as a risk factor for suicide
       among the elderly. The association of age and sex, however, is
       modified by sex, mental illness, and social relations. Men are more
       likely to commit suicide than women, as are people with mental
       illness and people who are widowed or divorced. During the past
       25 years, suicide rates for black men have tripled for an
       undetermined reason. Blazer recommends using risk factors to
       develop and improve suicide prevention interventions in the
       elderly population.

577   Brodaty, H., Harris, L., Peters, K., Wilhelm, K., Hickie, I., Boyce,
       P., Mitchell, P., Parker, G., & Eyers, K. (November, 1993).
       Prognosis of depression in the elderly: A comparison with
       younger patients. *British Journal of Psychiatry*, 163, 589-596.

The authors investigated the prognosis of depression in the elderly in a mixed-age sample of 242 consecutive referrals with DSM-III defined unipolar major depressive episode to a specialist unit for mood disorders. Subjects were followed-up at about 1 and 3.8 years. Analysis of the data found no significant difference in outcome between younger (ages 40 and under), middle aged (ages 40 to 59) and older (ages 60 and over) depressed patients. For the 61 elderly subjects with depression, prognosis improved with time, with 25% having a lasting recovery at the first and 41% at the second follow-up. Subjects with early-onset, recurrence, and poor premorbid personality had the worse prognosis for recovery. Three (5%) elderly depressives had committed suicide and seven (11%) had died from natural causes by the second follow-up. The authors concluded that there is a need for longer, more assertive treatment for elderly, depressed patients.

578   Canetto, Silvia Sara. (Spring, 1992). **Gender and suicide in the elderly**. *Suicide and Life-Threatening Behavior*, **22(1)**, 80-97.
The purpose of this article was to investigate the reasons why women are less vulnerable than men regarding suicide. The author summarizes findings from the literature related to epidemiology, physical factors, psychological factors, social and economic factors, and sociocultural factors. The author concludes that social and economic factors are not likely to account for older women's resilience. Neither do retirement and physical health factors. She hypothesizes that gender differences in suicide mortality reflect differences in coping and that women are more flexible and better able to accommodate and adapt to situations than men. They also have a greater capacity to be active, resourceful, and independent especially regarding personal care and socioemotional needs. They are more used to taking care of their households and often have a well-developed network of friends. She also concludes that women are influenced by gender norms regarding suicidal behavior. She proposes directions for developing prevention interventions which build on these findings.

579   Carpenter, Brian D. (June, 1993). **A review and new look at ethical suicide in advanced age**. *The Gerontologist*, *33*(3), 359-365.
This article is a review of theories of suicide and a summary of arguments against suicide. The author argues that the elderly have a unique claim to an ethical, unobstructed suicide based on

their developmental autonomy, which results from the experience and wisdom of the elderly.

580   Clark, David C. (Spring, 1993). Narcissistic crises of aging and suicidal despair. *Suicide and Life-Threatening Behavior*, 23(1), 21-26.

This review article describes some of the dangers inherent in oversimplifying the nature of suicide for public education purposes. The author outlines a model which he calls the "wedding-cake model" of elderly suicide which he derives from a community-based psychological autopsy study. The author hypothesizes that elderly persons who choose to die by suicide have a lifelong character fault that remains invisible until aging life changes force the issue into the open.

581   Cooper–Patrick, Lisa, Crum, Rosa M., & Ford, Daniel E. (December 14, 1994). Identifying suicidal ideation in general medical patients. *Journal of the American Medical Association*, 272(22), 1757-1762.

This article describes characteristics of general medical patients with suicidal ideation and presents a clinical strategy for identifying patients. Subjects were 6,041 people receiving care in a general medical setting over a six-month period. A total of 154 (2%) patients had experienced suicidal thoughts within the previous year. Data analysis identified the following characteristics as significantly related to having suicidal ideation: white relative to African American; separated or divorced relative to married; ages 18 to 30 or 31 to 50 versus those ages 65 and over. Gender, educational level, and socioeconomic status were not statistically associated. Psychiatric disorders significantly associated were major depression, panic disorder, alcohol disorder, and phobic disorder. Only 34% of the people with suicidal ideation met the criteria for major depression. A four-item screening instrument was developed to predict patients with suicidal ideation. Those items concerned symptoms of hopelessness, guilt, depressed mood, and sleep disturbances.

582   Edes, Thomas E. (January 19, 1994). Home visit. *Journal of the American Medical Association*, 271(3), 173.

This article presents a case study of an elderly man who is planning suicide and how the intervention of the doctor and a nurse saved a life.

583 Frierson, Robert L. (January, 1991). **Suicide attempts by the old and the very old.** *Archives of Internal Medicine, 151*(1), 141-144.

The author discusses the findings from a study of 95 patients between ages 60 and 90 who were evaluated by a psychiatric consultation service after a suicide attempt. Characteristics of this group included 1. a high degree of premeditation, 2. a tendency toward firearm use and wounds to the head, 3. male sex, 4. coexisting medical problems, 5. serious intent that increased by decade, 6. solitary living arrangements, 7. presence or history of a major psychiatric illness, and 8. ill health reported as a precipitant to suicidality. The most common psychiatric diagnosis was major depression. The most frequently observed physical ailments were congestive heart failure and chronic obstructive pulmonary disease. This population of attempters were similar to older persons who actually completed suicide. They were significantly different from a group of 1,630 attempters ages 16 to 59. The author recommends increased investigation of depressive features, treatment of alcohol abuse, early referral for psychiatric care, limited access to firearms, and strategies aimed at decreasing social isolation in order to decrease the likelihood of completed suicide in the elderly.

584 Glass, J. Conrad, Jr., & Reed, Susan E. (December, 1993). **To live or die: A look at elderly suicide.** *Educational Gerontology, 19*(8), 767-778.

This article is a discussion of characteristics of the elderly and factors which appear to be related to suicide. They point out that elderly people who attempt suicide seem to genuinely want to die rather than to be calling for help. They are more successful at suicide than those at other ages and use more lethal methods such as shooting and hanging. Women are more likely to use an overdose of sleeping pills. Researchers think that older people commit suicide as a response to losses and changes common in old age. Losses include social roles, health, strength and stamina, sensory losses, friends, and independence. Interventions that prevent suicide among the elderly must prevent the attempt. Verbal and behavioral clues must be observed. Support factors that can prevent suicide include providing financial resources, responding to clues, providing psychiatric counseling, and referring people to counseling when needed. The authors recommend increased public awareness of the problem and training for staff in recognizing suicide risk.

585   Gomberg, Edith S. Lisansky. (October, 1989). Suicide risk among women with alcohol problems. *American Journal of Public Health, 79*(10), 1363-1365.

This study reports suicide attempts in alcoholic and nonalcoholic women by age group. The subjects were 301 white women admitted to 21 alcoholism treatment facilities in Michigan and a sample of 137 nonalcoholic women matched for age and social class. The data showed a large difference between suicide attempts between the alcoholic (40%) and nonalcoholic (8.8%) women. Among alcoholic women, suicide attempts were twice as common at ages 20 to 29 as at ages 40 to 49. Alcoholic women also used significantly more nicotine, prescribed drugs, and banned substances.

586   Hendin, Herbert & Klerman, Gerald. (January, 1993). Physician– assisted suicide: The dangers of legalization. *American Journal of Psychiatry, 150*(1), 143-145.

The authors discuss physician-assisted suicide and explore the potential for abuse if legalization occurs. They discuss the reasons why older people may wish to die and how their fear of illness and depression puts them at risk of becoming victims. The authors discuss cases that have received public attention as examples of these abuses. They recommend that society's efforts should concentrate on providing treatment and relieving pain and helping individuals come to terms with death.

587   Horne, Amilda, & Blazer, Dan G. (February, 1992). The prevention of major depression in the elderly. *Clinics in Geriatric Medicine, 8*(1), 159-172.

This article discusses primary, secondary, and tertiary prevention of major depression in the elderly. The authors point out that conjugal bereavement is one of the most stressful life events and can lead to major depression. In one sample, 33% of recent widows could be diagnosed as clinically depressed. Another high-risk population is family caregivers of the cognitively impaired. They cite a study in which 40% of a population of caregivers were depressed. Primary prevention can include religious coping and social support. Decreasing prevalence of depression can also be accomplished with early intervention especially for people with Alzheimer's disease, Parkinson's disease, Huntington's disease, stroke, alcoholism, and severe medical illness. Long-term consequences of major depression such as suicide and alcoholism also can be addressed by prevention interventions. Clinicians should anticipate problems in people who have been depressed in the past, who are bereaved, in caretakers, and in patients with other illnesses and plan prevention or treatment.

588   Horton-Deutsch, Sara L., Clark, David C., & Farran, Carol J. (December, 1992). Chronic dyspnea and suicide in elderly men. *Hospital and Community Psychiatry, 43*(12), 1198-1203.

This study presents cases gathered from a community-based psychological autopsy that focused on elderly people who had completed suicide. The sample consisted of 73 cases of suicide by people ages 65 to 93 which occurred over a 10-month period. The researchers identified 14 men among the subjects whose chief complaint was chronic dyspnea. Each of these men had expressed concerns about their inability to breathe in the months or weeks before death. Of these 14 men, eight were married, four widowed, and two divorced. Death by gunshot wound was the most common method of suicide (n=10), followed by carbon monoxide intoxication (n=1) and falling from a high place (n=1). An analysis found that 13 had received a diagnosis of major depression, four had experienced problems with alcohol, four had lung cancer, and four had emphysema. The researchers point out the need for appropriate interventions for patients and families that will allow them to express their fear and suffering in some way other than suicide.

589   Humphry, Derek. (Spring, 1992). Rational suicide among the elderly. *Suicide and Life-Threatening Behavior, 22*(1), 125-129.

This paper outlines a perspective on elderly suicide that the author terms "voluntary euthanasia." He discusses the position of the Hemlock Society that suicide and assisted suicide should be ethically and legally acceptable for a person who is facing a terminal illness causing unbearable suffering. The author believes that legal euthanasia could extend, not shorten life, and reduce the number of suicides of elderly people since older people in good health would not fear a final illness in which there was no prospect for relief of suffering.

590   Kaplan, Mark S., Adamek, Margaret E., & Johnson, Scott. (February, 1994). Trends in firearm suicide among older American males: 1979-1988. *The Gerontologist, 34*(1), 59-65.

This article examines the incidence rates of firearm suicides for elderly males from 1979 through 1988. The authors examined data from the National Center for Health Statistics. They found that firearms were the most prevalent method of suicide for males and females. Males were six times more likely to use a firearm to commit suicide than females. Other methods used were poisoning, gas, car exhaust, hanging, and jumping. The authors believe that suicide is underreported on death certificates and so the true suicide rate may be underestimated. For older males, firearms are increasingly involved in suicide deaths among older Americans; elderly males showed the greatest proportional increase in the use of firearms as a method of suicide. The study did not address the question of whether limiting the availability of firearms would reduce elderly suicide; however, studies have shown that the presence of a firearm in the home increases the potential for violent death. The authors summarize several studies which show that more restrictive gun control laws reduce suicide rates in all age groups. They conclude that more attention must be directed toward the role of firearms in elderly suicide.

591   Kastenbaum, Robert. (Spring, 1992). Death, suicide and the older adult. *Suicide and Life-Threatening Behavior, 22*(1), 1-14.

This paper attempts to provide converging perspectives on death and suicide from the standpoints of both the external observer and the elderly person. Kastenbaum discusses implications derived from the elderly suicide data. He points out that morbidity and mortality increase with advancing adult age; that men are at greater risk for death across the life span; and that suicide is not a leading cause of death among older people as compared to other causes. In order to plan public policy, he recommends that policymakers consider the consequences of aging on older people. In the second part of the article, Kastenbaum discusses aging from the perspective of the older person. He discusses findings from studies of elderly people themselves which reveal a great diversity of attitudes toward death and concludes that stressful conditions of life arouse more anxiety among older people than does the prospect of death. Kastenbaum concludes with several suggestions for an ideal perspective on death and suicide in old age.

592   Lee, Melinda A., & Ganzini, Linda. (October, 1992). Depression in the elderly: Effect on patient attitudes toward life-sustaining therapy. *Journal of the American Geriatrics Society, 40*(10), 983-988.

The study examined the effect of depression on preferences for life-sustaining therapy in older persons. A survey comparing depressed, older veterans and a similar, but non-depressed, control group was conducted in a 490-bed Veterans Affairs teaching hospital. The subjects were medical inpatients ages 65 and over. Patients in intensive care, cognitively impaired, unable to communicate, abusing alcohol or drugs, or unable to return for outpatient care were excluded. Ninety-five eligible subjects (29%) refused to participate. Data were collected on 50 depressed and 50 control subjects using a self-administered questionnaire which assessed patients' preferences regarding life-saving interventions in their current state of health and in four hypothetical scenarios of serious illness. The researchers found that depressed subjects desired fewer interventions than control subjects in their current health and in hypothetical scenarios with a good prognosis (p ≤ .05). There were no differences between groups in poor prognosis scenarios. However, depression did not explain more than 5% of the decision-making variance in any situation. In good prognosis cases, subjects' quality of life assessment was the most powerful predictor of desire for life-saving interventions, accounting for 9% to 17% of the variance (p < .01). The authors concluded that depression is only a weak predictor of treatment refusal.

593 Lester, David, & Yang, Bijou. (1992). Social and economic correlates of the elderly suicide rate. *Suicide and Life-Threatening Behavior, 22*(1), 36-47.

This review of research examined regional studies, time-series studies, demographic shifts, and short-term impacts of suicide. They found that the suicide rates of the elderly show similar regional social correlates as the suicide rates of younger groups and that these rates can be explained using similar sociological theories. The time-series studies in the United States indicate that the impact of economic prosperity on the suicide rate of the elderly is beneficial, whereas the impact on the suicide rate of younger adults is detrimental. They conclude that social variables in the research they reviewed such as social isolation and divorce may be important in estimating elderly suicide risk.

594 Lobel, Brana, & Hirschfeld, Robert M. A. (1984). *Depression: What we know*. Rockville, MD: National Institute of Mental Health.

The authors describe clinical depression—what it is, who gets it, what causes it, and how to treat it. They point out that depressive symptoms are reported by almost 20% of elderly; however, the true incidence and prevalence of clinical depression are not known. They note also that a third of the suicides are committed by people ages 55 and over and that a large percentage of suicides are committed by people who are clinically depressed.

595   Loebel, J. Pierre, Loebel, Justine S., Dager, Stephen R., Centerwall, Brandon S., & Reay, Donald T. (April, 1991). Anticipation of nursing home placement may be a precipitant of suicide among the elderly. *Journal of the American Geriatrics Society, 39*(4), 407-408.

This study investigated a group of 57 people ages 65 to 92 who had committed suicide in 1986. The group consisted of 43 males and 14 females (mean age 74.4 years), 25 (44%) of whom were married. Researchers found that of the 18 who gave reasons for their suicide in notes or comments to informants, 8 (44%) said their suicide was motivated by anticipation of nursing home placement. Other factors were depression, chronic or painful illness. The average age of this subgroup was 78.1. There were six males and two females; all were Caucasian; five (63%) were married, two were widowed, and one divorced. The investigators then examined the possible influence of marital status on fear of nursing home placement with a group of 30 married elderly persons living in a retirement home matched with the original group for age and gender. The majority (58%) cited physical health as their major concern; 34% had mental health concerns; and 10% cited fear of a need for nursing home placement. Data analysis found that married persons were more likely to fear nursing home placement than unmarried persons (p < .05). The authors suggest that health care providers plan for nursing home placement cautiously, especially when dealing with married individuals.

596   Lyness, Jeffrey M., Conwell, Yeates, & Nelson, J. Craig. (April, 1992). Suicide attempts in elderly psychiatric inpatients. *Journal of the American Geriatrics Society, 40*(4), 320-324.

This study investigated psychopathological characteristics of elderly suicide attempters who had been admitted to an inpatient psychiatric unit. Subjects were patients ages 60 and over treated at the unit between 1979 and 1984. Of the 168 patients, 25 had made a suicide attempt. The most common method was medication overdose. Other methods were ingestion of poisons, lacerations, strangulation, carbon monoxide poisoning, hanging, and jumping. The investigators found that 80% of the attempters had a major depressive syndrome; among those with affective disorders, age was significantly related to attempts. Substance abuse and dementia were uncommon diagnoses.

597 McIntosh, John L. (Spring, 1992). Epidemiology of suicide in the elderly. *Suicide and Life-Threatening Behavior,* 22(1), 15-35.
　　　This article is a discussion of current levels and trends regarding suicide among the elderly in the United States. McIntosh details age, sex, race, marital status, and methods of suicide as factors in suicide among the old and discusses past trends and future predictions of changes in elderly suicide rates. In addition to fatal suicidal behaviors, he presents data and literature on parasuicide and survivors of elderly suicide.

598 Meeham, Patrick J., Saltzman, Linda E., & Sattin, Richard W. (September, 1991). Suicides among older United States residents: Epidemiologic characteristics and trends. *American Journal of Public Health,* 81(9), 1198-1200.
　　　This report discusses data concerning suicide deaths compiled by the National Center for Health Statistics. A total of 36,789 suicides were reported among United States residents ages 65 and over during 1980 to 1986. White elderly men had the highest suicide rate, followed by black men, white women, and black women. During the study period, the suicide rate increased 23% in white men, 42% in black men, and 17% in white women. Divorced men were three times more likely to commit suicide than married men and nearly 19 times more likely than married women. The suicide rate for divorced men increased 38%. The most common method of suicide for men and women ages 65 and over was firearms (65%). The use of drugs and poisons was a common method for elderly women. Depression, alcoholism, and chronic illnesses are known risk factors for suicide. The authors suggest that the problem of social isolation in the elderly may be an important issue to address as a prevention strategy. Factors related to social disruption (death of spouse, divorce, relocation) are also important.

599 Moody, Harry R. (1991). "Rational suicide" on grounds of old age? *Journal of Geriatric Psychiatry,* 24(2), 261-276.
　　　The author discusses the issue of suicide as a choice for older people who are too sick or frail to maintain an acceptable quality of life. This question is invited, says Moody, by increasing morbidity at the same time mortality is declining. He argues that

suicide should be recognized as a serious and legitimate solution
to problems of aging.

600   Motto, Jerome A. (Spring, 1991). **An integrated approach to
estimating suicide risk.** *Suicide and Life-Threatening Behavior,*
21(1), 74–89.

This article describes the complex issues involved in the
assessment of suicide risk. Even the most accurate assessment,
used as a tool to direct treatment, does not necessarily guarantee
successful intervention or outcome. The author uses five case
histories to illustrate the methods and problems of suicide risk
assessment.

601   Nieto, Evaristo, Vieta, E., Lázaro, L., Gastó, C., & Cirera, E. (July,
1992). **Serious suicide attempts in the elderly.** *Psychopathology,*
25(4), 183–188.

This study investigated specific characteristics of nonfatal
serious suicidal behavior among the elderly population. The 257
patients studied were selected from 4,850 patients seen in a
psychiatric unit during a 6-year period because they had
attempted suicide. The main diagnosis of the attempters was major
depression (68.3%). The most common methods were self-
poisoning with drugs or other substances, and single cuts in the
arm. Other methods included jumping, hanging, shooting, and
piercing. The 38 attempters ages 65 and over accounted for 14.8%
of those who made serious suicide attempts. The authors found
that the elderly used more lethal methods than younger
attempters. None of the elderly were suffering from delirium or
dementia prior to the suicidal act. Since 75% of the elderly suffered
from an affective disorder, the authors concluded that nonfatal
serious suicidal behavior in the elderly is generally the result of a
clinically significant and treatable affective disorder not attributed
to physical illness, loneliness, or age. Physicians and psychiatrists
need to be trained to diagnose and treat depression.

602   Osgood, Nancy J. (1987). **The alcohol/suicide connection in later
life.** *Postgraduate Medicine, 81*(4), 379–384.

The many losses and stresses of late life, often accompanied
by feelings of loneliness and depression, make the elderly
especially vulnerable to alcoholism and suicide. The elderly
alcoholic is at significant risk for suicide. The major factors in
geriatric alcoholism and suicide are depression (manifested by
changes in sleeping and eating patterns, somatic complaints, and

apathy), stress and loss, and helplessness and hopelessness. Alcoholism in the elderly can be detected and effectively treated, thus reducing the risk of suicide. Family and friends, physicians, and society all have a role in preventing alcoholism in the elderly.

603 **Osgood, Nancy J. (1991). Prevention of suicide in the elderly.** *Journal of Geriatric Psychiatry,* 24(2), 293-307.
This article presents a discussion of the prevalence of suicide among the elderly and possible risk factors. The author discusses the need for education and training among caregivers and professionals who encounter depressed suicidal elderly. She discusses several myths associated with suicide which should be dispelled by education. She points out that older adults give clues prior to their act, they are serious about committing suicide when they discuss the topic, and unlike younger people, they do not use suicidal threats to gain attention or manipulate others. She also describes high-risk groups, especially elderly, white, single males, alcoholics, depressed adults, those living alone and socially isolated, and the recently bereaved. Osgood describes a variety of techniques and strategies for prevention, early detection, and treatment of depressed and suicidal elderly. She concludes that suicide among the elderly is preventable through education, training, early detection, treatment, expansion and development of health services, and restriction of firearms.

604 **Osgood, Nancy J. (1992). Environmental factors in suicide in long-term care facilities.** *Suicide and Life-threatening Behavior,* 22(1), 98-106.
This study identified environmental factors related to suicide in long-term care facilities. Questionnaires were mailed to a random sample of administrators at 1,080 facilities. Information was collected on facility characteristics, overt suicide, and intentional life-threatening behavior. The study sample consisted of 463 returned questionnaires. Total resident population represented was 30,269, ranging in age from 22 to 91 (mean age 65 years). Of the respondents, 84 facilities reported at least one suicide. Chi-square analyses revealed four-environmental characteristics related to suicidal behavior and deaths from suicide: staff turnover, size, auspices, and per diem cost. More suicides occurred in larger facilities and facilities with higher staff turnover. Religious or "other" facilities experienced more suicidal deaths than public or private facilities; facilities charging less experienced more deaths.

605   Osgood, Nancy J. (1992). *Suicide in later life: Recognizing the warning signs.* New York: Lexington Books.

This book discusses various losses associated with aging which are related to suicide and why some people commit suicide and others do not. The author explores the alcohol-suicide connection and presents warning signs and suggestions for prevention. Among the components of a prevention program are maintaining physical health (eating well, keeping fit to reduce stress), social health, and emotional health. She also discusses spiritual health. The author concludes the book with a discussion of the right to die and presents a case against eldercide.

606   Osgood, Nancy J. (1992). Suicide in the elderly: Etiology and assessment. *International Review of Psychiatry, 4,* 217-223.

This article discusses several issues related to suicide among the elderly. The suicide rate in the United States for those ages 65 and over is 50% higher than the rate for teenagers or the national rate. The author points out that the majority of older adults use a gun to commit suicide. She states that self-starvation and refusal of life-sustaining medications are the most common methods of suicide among residents in nursing homes and other long term care facilities. Most at-risk are males, caucasians, recently widowed, and people ages 75 and over. Other risk factors are aging-related loss and stress, depression, and alcoholism. Accurate diagnosis and assessment strategies and techniques highlighted in the article include: diagnostic interview, physical examination, laboratory tests, history taking, and rating scales.

607   Osgood, Nancy J., Brant, Barbara A., & Lipman, Aaron. (1991). *Suicide among the elderly in long term care facilities.* Westport, CT: Greenwood Press.

This book presents a comprehensive overview to the topic of elderly suicide as well as the findings of a study of suicide in long-term care facilities. The authors discuss issues related to prevalence, risk factors, and prevention. The authors recommend identifying and treating depression as one important primary prevention effort. They recommend that nursing staff and other elderly caregivers receive training in recognizing clues and warning signs of depression and suicidal intentions.

608   Osgood, Nancy J., & Eisenhandler, Susan A. (Spring, 1994). Gender and assisted and acquiescent suicide: A suicidologist's perspective. *Issues in Law & Medicine, 9*(4), 361-374.

This article discusses ethical and legal issues related to assisted suicide and acquiescent suicide. They present the cases of Janet Adkins and Dr. Kevorkian and Emily Gilbert as examples. The authors point out that the majority of assisted suicide cases involve middle-aged women. They also point out cases where women have participated in murder-suicide pacts even though they were not ill themselves because they could not bear to live without their husbands. They also discuss acquiescent suicide, a form that occurs in relatively isolated settings such as institutions and present a detailed case study. Acquiescent suicide is accomplished by refusing food, medications, and social interactions primarily due to the hopelessness of their situations. The authors call for education and enlightenment of people about gender issues and suicide.

609   Parmelee, Patricia A., Katz, Ira R., & Lawton, M. Powell. (1989). **Depression among the institutionalized aged: Assessment and prevalence estimation.** *Journals of Gerontology, 44*(1), M22-M29.

This study screened nursing home and congregate residents at a large residential facility for the aged for symptoms of depression and cognitive impairment. Of 708 survey respondents, 12.4% met DSM-III-R criteria for major depression. About half of those suffering depression also had significant cognitive deficits. Another 30.5% reported less severe depression. Residents of the congregate living units displayed lower levels of depression and significantly less cognitive impairment than residents of the nursing home. Major depression was more common among the persons recently admitted to the facility than among long-term residents. Long-term residents were more likely to display cognitive deficits in combination with minor depression. The authors conclude that depression is a major problem among elderly in residential care settings including the relatively healthy, active residents of congregate facilities. On the positive side, symptoms of depression can be assessed by trained nonprofessionals who can identify those who may need clinical intervention.

610   Richardson, Roberta, Lowenstein, Steven, & Weissberg, Michael. (September, 1989). **Coping with the suicidal elderly: A physician's guide.** *Geriatrics, 44*(9), 43-47, 51.

This article presents guidance to physicians to assist them in identifying and treating elderly people considering suicide. Many older people visit a physician shortly before they commit suicide thus presenting the physician with an opportunity to intervene. The authors include a profile of the suicidal elderly and discuss major risk factors that physicians should look for which may signal a risk of suicide such as depression, recent losses, bereavement, psychiatric illnesses, and chronic medical illness. Several management options and therapies are presented for consideration. Physicians must act decisively in recognition of the fact that suicidality is a transient, treatable condition.

611   Rifai, A. H., Reynolds, C. F., & Mann, J. J. (1992). Biology of elderly suicide. *Suicide and Life-Threatening Behavior*, 22(1), 48-61.

This review describes normal aging effects on the central nervous system pertinent to the biology of suicide and then reviews port-mortem biological studies of the brains of suicides and suicide attempters. Post-mortem studies of suicide victims and suicide attempters were analyzed. Also reviewed are biological studies of aggression and impulsivity. Finally, the authors describe data on the effect of degenerative diseases on the serotonin system and the possible link to increased suicidal behavior in affected patients. While various biological parameters have been found to correlate with suicidal behavior, most studies have not included a meaningful number of subjects ages 60 and over. The authors point out the need for further study of the biology of suicide in the geriatric age group.

612   Rodin, Gary, & Voshart, Karen. (June, 1986). Depression in the medically ill: An overview. *American Journal of Psychiatry*, 143(6), 696-705.

This study reviewed the literature on the association between depression and medical illness in order to provide a clinical perspective on the problem. The authors found that depression is common among the medically ill and may occur in association with or as part of the individual response to the illness. Blurred boundaries and overlap make it difficult for physicians to distinguish between depression as a symptom and as a clinical syndrome. The biological mechanisms underlying depressive disorders are poorly understood in medical patients as in other patients with depression. Medical illness, however, may be a significant psychosocial stressor because of its potential impact on psychological and social functioning, the ability to work, maintain roles, and sustain self-esteem. Antidepressant medications may be helpful in depressed medically ill patients but additional controlled studies are needed.

613 Rosowsky, Erlene. (Winter, 1993). Suicidal behavior in the nursing home and a postsuicide intervention. *American Journal of Psychotherapy, 47*(1), 127-142.

This article presents a case history of an elderly suicidal patient and a review of current literature on elderly suicide. Topics included in the literature review are epidemiology, risk factors (losses, medical factors, mental illness, personality), and suicide risk in long-term care facilities. The author discusses the effect of institutionalization and relocation as a catalyst for suicide. Suicidal ideation, response to suicide, and postsuicide intervention process are discussed in depth. Using the case study, Rosowsky points out how risk factors manifested themselves and should have sent signals to the family and staff. The author concludes that the training needs of the primary care physician should be addressed in order to diagnose and medically intervene when necessary. The article concludes with a model of suicide probability in the nursing home resident including risks, stressors, catalysts, and context.

614 Schmid, Hermann, Manjee, Kim, & Shah, Tulshi. (June, 1994). On the distinction of suicide ideation versus attempt in elderly psychiatric inpatients. *The Gerontologist, 34*(3), 332-339.

The purpose of this study was to differentiate risk factors for suicidal ideation versus attempt. Ideators were defined as seriously thinking about, wishing, or planning suicide. Attempters were defined as any person with a history of serious self-inflicted harm with suicidal intent. The subjects were 93 female and 59 male elderly patients ages 59 to 89 (mean age 69.6 years). Their chief complaints were depression and new onset suicide attempt or suicidal ideation. Of the total group, 97 were attempters. Methods were drug overdose (51.5%), combined drug-alcohol overdose (12.4%), alcohol (8.2%), deep cutting or stabbing (12.4%), hanging (8.2%), firearms (3.1%), drowning (2.1%), and jumping from heights (2.1%). Data analysis identified several significant predictors of suicide attempt versus ideation. Elderly at greater risk for attempt were Protestant, living at home, neat by appearance and calm in behavior at admission, and currently being treated with antianxiety or antipsychotic medication. Elderly at greater risk for ideation were Catholic or Jewish, living in nursing homes and disorderly in appearance and behavior at admission, and not on antianxiety or antipsychotic medication.

Among the sociodemographic variables, living arrangement was the most significant variable. Elderly individuals living in nursing homes were far less likely to be attempters than those not institutionalized regardless of whether they were living alone, with a spouse or with children. With respect to mental status, ideators had higher scores than attempters in terms of disorderly appearance and thought disorganization. The authors commented that the established risk factors for suicide completion (male, widowed, divorced, isolated, physically ill) did not appear to be significant in distinguishing attempters from ideators.

615   Smith-Stoner, Marilyn. (March, 1994). Suicide and the elderly: Can the LP/VN help? *The Journal of Practical Nursing,* 44(1), 36-41.

This article discusses common myths concerning suicide and the elderly; factors leading to the elderly person's feeling that life has no meaning; the relationship between alcoholism, depression, and suicide; and interventions that an LP/VN can do to assist depressed clients. The author points out ways that elderly suicide differs from youth suicide. Elderly people use guns, are more likely to be successful in their first attempt, often exhibit no warning signs, are well planned, and are often committed by people with a chronic disease. This article includes a multiple choice exam and answer key and is appropriate for use as in-service training.

616   Strasburger, Larry H., & Welpton, Sue S. (1991). Elderly suicide: Minimizing risk for patient and professional. *Journal of Geriatric Psychiatry,* 224(2), 235-259.

This literature review presents a thorough overview of the problem of elderly suicide along with several case studies. The authors identify risk factors as: previous attempts, family history of suicide, male, white race, recent losses (financial, roles, change in environment, relationships), anniversary of a loss, loss of ability to cope, physical illnesses, psychiatric disorder. They recommend a mental examination as part of every assessment of an elderly person. They present comprehensive suggestions for treatment and management and minimizing professional risk. The authors conclude that elderly suicide will continue to be a prominent problem producing complex and tragic results. Clinicians need to cope more effectively with this issue.

617 Valente, Sharon M. (1993-1994). Suicide and elderly people: Assessment and intervention. *Omega, 28*(4), 317-332.

This article presents a detailed case study to illustrate risk assessment, interventions, and outcomes. The subject was an elderly woman whose depression with low suicide risk initially responded well to outpatient treatment. She subsequently became highly suicidal after her husband's death. The author details types of communication that present verbal cues of suicidal intent. She also includes a comprehensive plan for risk assessment and interventions.

618 Weishaar, Marjorie E., & Beck, Aaron T. (1990). Cognitive approaches to understanding and treating suicidal behavior. In Susan J. Blumenthal, & David J. Kupfer (Eds.), *Suicide over the life cycle: Risk factors, assessment, and treatment of suicidal patients* (pp. 469-477). Washington, DC: American Psychiatric Press, Inc.

This chapter discusses three assessment instruments developed by Aaron Beck to assist in the systematic evaluation of an individual's suicidality. The Scale for Suicide Ideation is a 19-item instrument which assesses suicide intention. The Suicide Intent Scale is used with patients who have attempted suicide and evaluates the severity of the patient's psychological intent at the time of the attempt. The Hopelessness Scale is a 20-item instrument to which the individuals respond true or false to each item which has a moderately high correlation with the Beck Depression Inventory and with clinical ratings of hopelessness. Hopelessness is more strongly related to suicidal intent than depression. Copies of the instruments are included in the appendices.

619 What's new: Gallup survey: Physicians need to detect suicide warning signs. (April, 1993). *Geriatrics, 48*(4), 16.

This article reports the results of a Gallup survey that suggests many suicides could be prevented if primary care physicians were to detect the warning signs of depression and properly treat it. The survey polled 802 Americans ages 60 and over who lived independently. One percent had thought of committing suicide within the last six months and 6% knew of someone else ages 60 and over who had attempted suicide. During their last physical examination only 6% had been asked about depression or suicide ideation by their physicians. More than one-fourth reported that suicide was a personal decision and others shouldn't be involved.

620   **Zweig, Richard A., & Hinrichsen, Gregory A. (November, 1993). Factors associated with suicide attempts by depressed older adults: A prospective study.** *American Journal of Psychiatry,* *150*(11), 1687-1692.

This study investigated demographic, clinical, and interpersonal factors prospectively associated with suicide attempts by older adults with major depressive disorder. The researchers administered a structured diagnostic interview to elderly inpatients diagnosed as having major depressive disorder according to the Research Diagnostic Criteria. Subjects were followed-up for one year. Elderly patients who attempted suicide during the follow-up period were compared with the nonattempters across demographic, clinical, and interpersonal factors assessed during the initial interviews. A suicide attempt was made by 8.7% (N=11) of the 126 elderly depressed patients within one year after hospital admission. Compared with nonattempters, attempters were of a higher socioeconomic status, had more past suicide attempts and current suicidal behavior, and made up a disproportionately large percentage of those patients who had never had a remission of their index depressive episodes. Spouses and adult children of patients who later attempted suicide evidenced more psychiatric symptoms, more strain in the relative-patient relationship, and more difficulties in caring for the patient than the relatives of nonattempters. The authors stressed the need for careful attention to both clinical and interpersonal factors in the assessment of suicide risk in the elderly.

Author Index

Entries are keyed to page numbers.

A

M

Parham, Iris A., 53
Parker, G., 260
Parkinson, Michael D., 5
Parmelee, Patricia A., 273
Parrish, Gib, 4
Pascaru, Adina, 150
Patriarca, Peter A., 164, 165
Paveza, Gregory J., 107, 229
Payette, Helene, 188
Payne, Barbara P., 58, 223, 230, 235
Pearlman, Cindy, 137
Peck, William A., 121, 131, 209
Peddecord, K. Michael, 51
Pendergast, David R., 125
Pendergast, Jane F., 219
Pentland, Brian, 138
Perlman, Gary D., 245
Perrone, Jeanmarie, 172
Persson, Diane, 249
Pestle, Ruth E., 160
Peters, K., 260
Petersen, David M., 58, 223, 230, 235
Petersen, M. M., 131
Petraglia, John S., 71
Phillips, Jim, 142
Phyland, Debra J., 78
Pillemer, Karl A., 94, 102, 107, 108, 109, 113
Pinel, Carl, 173
Platt, J. S., 47
Plichta, Denise T., 213
Plueckhahn, Vernon D., 90, 91
Poddig, Barbara, 228
Poff, Gregory A., 223
Polito, A., 187
Pollow, Rachel L., 35, 224
Popkin, Barry M., 179
Powell, Lynda, 145
Powell, Sharon, 109
Press, Edward, 91
Pressler, R., 170

Pritchard, Jacki, 110

Q

Quinn, Mary Joy, 110

R

Rammohan, Meenakshi, 197
Ranaldi, L., 187
Rapoport, Yoram, 86
Rasmussen, Reva, 58
Ray, Wayne A., 249, 250
Rearden, John J., 247
Reay, Donald T., 268
Reed, A. Thomas, 131
Reed, Susan E., 263
Reeves, Robert D., 218
Reichman, William E., 97
Remington, Patrick L., 253
Repasy, Andrew, 162
Resnick, Neil M., 126
Retchin, Sheldon M., 250, 256
Reynolds, C. F., 274
Rhyne, Robert, 20
Rice, Dorothy, 11
Richardson, Roberta, 273
Richman, Donna, 145
Ried, L. Douglas, 224
Rifai, A. H., 274
Riley, Mary Ellen, 84
Rimm, Alfred A., 21, 129
Rivara, Frederick P., 116
Rivera, Patricia, 101
Robbins, A. S., 173
Robbins, Alan S., 139
Robbins, Lee N., 45
Roberts, Pamela C., 251
Roberts, W. Neal, 251
Robertson, Leon S., 11, 238
Robinson, Elizabeth G., 135
Robinson, Nell B., 81
Robinson-Hawkins, Susan, 122

Subject Index

Entries are keyed to page numbers.

E

About the Compiler

BONNIE L. WALKER is president of Bonnie Walker & Associates, Inc., in Crofton, Maryland. She has been the principal investigator for several grants funded by the National Institutes of Health including: Fire Safety for the Elderly (NIA), Drug Prevention Materials for African American Patients (NIAAA), Screening the Elderly for Problem Use of Alcohol (NIAAA), Injury Prevention for the Elderly (CDC and NIA), and Injury Prevention for Young Children (CDC). She has also been the principal investigator for two grants from DHHS: Fire Safety for Board and Care Operators and Independent Living Skills for Older Youth in Foster Care. Walker has been on the faculties of Bowie State University, Gallaudet University, and Trinity College.

ISBN 0-313-29670-7

90000>

EAN

9 780313 296703

HARDCOVER BAR CODE